BLACK HEALTH
LIBRARY GUIDE

OBESITY

BLACK HEALTH LIBRARY GUIDE

OBESITY

Vital Health Information for African Americans

Mavis Thompson, M.D.
with Kirk A. Johnson

Edited by Linda Villarosa
Nutritional Advisor, Maudene Nelson
Illustrated by Marcelo Oliver

KENSINGTON BOOKS
KENSINGTON PUBLISHING CORP.
http://www.kensingtonbooks.com

This book is not intended as a substitute for medical advice of physicians and should be used only in conjunction with the advice of your personal doctor. The reader should regularly consult a physician in matters relating to his or her health and particularly with respect to any symptoms that may require diagnosis or medical attention.

KENSINGTON BOOKS are published by

Kensington Publishing Corp.
850 Third Avenue
New York, NY 10022

First Kensington Printing: December, 1999
10 9 8 7 6 5 4 3 2 1

Printed in the United States of America

For the millions of overweight black Americans who are finding new joy by caring for their health.

Contents

Contents

Foreword

Being overweight has never been easy. Ostracized at school and work, ridiculed in public, fat people have always had to work a little harder to win courtesies and rights that thin folks take for granted. And those of us who are heavy and black know the unique challenges that brown skin and ample bodies bring in a society geared to whites who are thin.

But change is in the air. Throughout the United States, fat people are leading a revolution. In a drive that shadows the civil rights battles of the 1960s, the "fat acceptance" movement is spreading its call for equality, acceptance, freedom, and self-respect.

Medical advances are bringing change, too. More than ever before, doctors are finding surprising answers to the riddle of why some people are heavier than others, and why African-Americans, particularly females, are among the heaviest people in the country.

And medical researchers are redefining what constitutes "healthy" body weight, a change that gives African-Americans the best benchmark we've ever had to judge whether our weight may be hurting our health.

Change has even come to the generations-old struggle to lose weight. That's because researchers tell us that, contrary to popular belief, diets don't work. In fact, diets can actually make you *gain* weight. But there *is* a medically accepted path to permanent weight loss. That's important news for black folks concerned about their health and their waistlines.

These are just a few of the important topics covered in this *Guide to Obesity*. It's a book that interweaves the latest medical findings with frank talk about how African-Americans are coming to peace with our body weight, and learning to live fuller, more joyous lives.

Chapter 1 ("Blacks and Obesity: An Introduction") defines obesity, discusses its prevalence in the black community, and explains why body weight poses special challenges to African-Americans.

Chapter 2 ("What's So Bad About Being Fat?") contrasts the modern obsession with thinness with the growing movement for fat acceptance. In straightforward language, it discusses the health risks that excess weight brings African-Americans, describing a simple test to help you determine if the *location* of your body fat may cause a health hazard. It also discusses the special emotional challenges of being overweight and black, and how discrimination against fat people can present hurdles that thin people can only imagine.

Chapter 3 ("What Makes People Obese?") reveals how a person's body weight is related to income, education, eating habits, and a number of other social and environmental factors, including child abuse. It also discusses new evidence that body weight may be determined by genetic triggers, and other biological factors that lie beyond our control.

Chapter 4 ("The Truth About Dieting") reveals the one fact that diet plans and weight-loss centers never tell you: diets don't work because your body's ability to slow your metabolism works as built-in protection against starvation.

If diets won't do the job, what will? It takes a change in lifestyle, which includes a combination of eating right *and* exercising. Chapter 5 ("The 'E' Word: An Important and Neglected Ally") explains how exercise fits into the picture, and how little weight many African-Americans actually have to lose in order to feel better and be healthier.

Chapter 6 ("If Dieting Doesn't Work, What Should I Eat?") takes a look at why African-Americans eat what we do, and how you can construct a personal eating plan that features sensible food choices without sacrificing taste. The trick is to redefine your relationship with food by using success-tested hints and strategies that make your food choices work for you. Chapter 6 also features a sure-fire weight-reduction program endorsed by the author.

Chapter 7 ("Helping Our Kids Fight Fat") explains why we should pay attention to obesity among African-American children, and how we can help our kids grow up healthy and fit despite an onslaught of TV commercials for greasy pizza and sugary breakfast cereals.

Chapter 8 ("Menus for Healthful Weight Loss") shows you how easy it is to prepare meals using the guidelines presented in this book. The chapter also provides handy information on the nutrient content of common foods.

The book is written in a friendly, conversational style, and you don't need a background in medicine or science to understand it. It's a hopeful book, one intended to inspire you and encourage you to be happy and at peace with your body, regardless of your weight. Here's hoping these pages help you move down the road to health and wholeness.

M.T. New York, New York
K.J. Champaign, Illinois
February 1999

CHAPTER 1

Blacks and Obesity: An Introduction

Imagine an epidemic that affects nearly one in three African-Americans, sends millions to the hospital and others to an early grave, but whose effects can be minimized by anyone at any age at any time at virtually no cost.

That's the best way to describe obesity: It's a problem and it's a mystery. The problem is that being heavy often comes linked with profound challenges to our physical and emotional well-being—challenges that make fatness and blackness a unique and often difficult combination. The mystery is what to do about it—how to lose weight and keep it off; how to be at peace with our bodies; how to make friends with food; how to feel good about ourselves in a culture that, for all black people but especially those of us who are large, strews roadblocks in the path of our self-esteem.

By all accounts, we're becoming a nation of heavyweights—and that worries doctors. A whopping 97 million Americans age twenty to seventy-four are either overweight or obese. That's a bit more than half of all adults coast to coast. In other words, Americans of "normal" weight or under are in the minority.

Obesity is particularly prevalent in the black community. Over 30 percent of all African-Americans are obese. In fact, black women are among the heaviest of all Americans. Nationwide, around 52 percent of all black women are obese, compared to 33 percent of all white women. A few years ago, Minister Abdul Alim Muhammad, M.D., of the Nation of Islam released a report showing that although the average female member of the Nation was obese, and the average male was overweight, members were probably still healthier than African-Americans as a whole. In Dr. Mohammad's view, that can only mean one thing: "We as a people are in serious trouble."

Being fat poses special challenges for black Americans. For one thing, black folks are disproportionately poor. And while overweight is slightly less prevalent in low-income men as compared to men above the poverty level, it's nearly twice as common in low-income women compared to their more affluent sisters. So in women, at least, poverty seems to present black people with certain conditions that increase the probability of obesity.

The black community also suffers an inordinate amount of serious illness and disease, which can compound the effects of excess weight. Being fat predisposes us to a number of diseases, including heart disease, diabetes, and hypertension. Black Americans have staggeringly high rates of these diseases to begin with, because of our genes and our lifestyle. So African-Americans who are heavy face a double whammy—from two directions we run a significant risk of developing debilitating and even life-threatening illness.

In addition, obesity can place black Americans in the awkward position of facing discrimination by both whites and blacks. If you are overweight and black, you learn at an early age that fatness is one of our culture's most enduring taboos. It gives whites license to discriminate when they wouldn't dare bother someone whose skin is just as black but who weighs less, and it can spoil alliances with other blacks who have bought into the prevailing distaste for plumpness. Dr. E. K. Daufin, an assistant professor at California State University at Los Angeles, says the problem is a double standard. "When someone called me the N word—meaning I was lazy, ugly, stupid and subhuman—my parents taught me to defend myself against the nasty epithet. They taught me to have dignity in the face of racial slurs because they were, my parents assured me, false," Daufin explained to the *Los Angeles Times*. "But when someone called me 'fat'—meaning I was lazy, ugly, undisciplined, and an interior human—my parents taught me to acquiesce in the face of what, they assured me, was the truth."

These are just several of the many reasons that, while obese blacks have much in common with obese whites, body size presents African-Americans with an entirely different layer of difficult, complex issues. Dick Gregory realized that when he called on Congress to establish a new branch of the National Institutes of Health called the National Institute of Obesity and Weight Management. The comedian-turned-activist-turned-diet-consultant suggested the idea, with backing from the Congressional Black Caucus, in light of the huge numbers of black Americans who weigh more than the supposed ideal (Gregory once weighed 350 pounds himself; he discovered fasting during political protests), and because of the present gaps in what researchers know about black obesity. Though Gregory's suggestion was never incorporated into a bill, its backing by some of the most powerful African-American political leaders underscores both the seriousness of black obesity and the extent to which the issue has not been fully addressed by health researchers.

What is obesity, exactly? We may know it when we see it (or feel it). To most of us, it means girth and heft: thick thighs, heavy hips, substantial stomachs. It's about tape measures and bathroom scales and frustration and hope. But is there a more universal definition?

As it turns out, there is. For a long time, doctors have used height-weight tables to figure out if a person is overweight. You may have seen these charts; based on insurance-industry data, they give so-called ideal weights for men and women based on their height.

Nowadays doctors use a different—and better—measure to tell whether a person's weight falls in the healthy range. They use something called a body-mass index, or BMI. Now, the BMI may sound like a fancy car, but it's got nothing at all to do with a BMW. It's one number that takes into account both your height and weight. To estimate your BMI, find your height in the left column. Then find your weight along the top row. Your BMI is where the row and column intersect.

Uncle Sam says the healthiest BMIs range from 19 to 24.9. In fact, the ideal BMI, for men at least, may be around 22. That's the number associated with the lowest risk of diabetes, stroke, and coronary heart disease in a recent large-scale study of men in Great Britain. For women, an ideal BMI is slightly less than it is for men.

Key: 25–29.9: overweight
30 and above: obese

Height	*Weight*										
	100	105	110	115	120	125	130	135	140	145	150
5'0"	20	21	22	23	23	24	25	26	27	28	29
5'1"	19	20	21	22	23	24	25	26	26	27	28
5'2"	18	19	20	21	22	23	24	25	26	27	28
5'3"	18	19	20	20	21	22	23	24	25	26	27
5'4"	17	18	19	20	21	22	22	23	24	25	26
5'5"	17	18	18	19	20	21	22	22	23	24	25
5'6"	16	17	18	19	19	20	21	22	23	24	24
5'7"	16	17	17	18	19	20	20	21	22	23	24
5'8"	15	16	17	18	18	19	20	21	21	22	23
5'9"	15	16	16	17	18	19	19	20	21	22	22
5'10"	14	15	16	17	17	18	19	19	20	21	22
5'11"	14	15	15	16	17	18	18	19	20	20	21
6'0"	14	14	15	16	16	17	18	18	19	20	20
6'1"	13	14	15	15	16	17	17	18	19	19	20
6'2"	13	14	14	15	15	16	17	17	18	19	19

Height	*Weight*										
	155	160	165	170	175	180	185	190	195	200	205
5'0"	30	31	32	33	34	35	36	37	38	39	40
5'1"	29	30	31	32	33	34	35	36	37	38	39
5'2"	28	29	30	31	32	33	34	35	36	37	37
5'3"	28	28	29	30	31	32	33	34	35	36	36
5'4"	27	28	28	29	30	31	32	33	34	34	35
5'5"	26	27	28	28	29	30	31	32	33	33	34
5'6"	25	26	27	28	28	29	30	31	32	32	33
5'7"	24	25	26	27	28	28	29	30	31	31	32
5'8"	24	24	25	26	27	27	28	29	30	31	31
5'9"	23	24	24	25	26	27	27	28	29	30	30
5'10"	22	23	24	24	25	26	27	27	28	29	30
5'11"	22	22	23	24	25	25	26	26	27	28	29
6'0"	21	22	22	23	24	25	25	26	26	27	28
6'1"	21	21	22	23	23	24	25	25	26	26	27
6'2"	20	21	21	22	23	23	24	24	25	26	26

If your BMI is 25 to 29.9, consider yourself *overweight.* If it's 30 or higher, then you're considered *obese.* Regardless of which category you may fall into, hear this: If you're hefty and you're black, you should take your weight very seriously. Although not every overweight African-American is in poor health, millions of us have weight-related illnesses. And millions others who may seem perfectly healthy are at higher risk of serious and sometimes fatal diseases. If you're fat but not presently sick, losing weight can decrease your risk of becoming ill down the road. And if you're struggling today with hypertension, diabetes, joint problems, and other weight-related diseases, take heart, because losing weight often diminishes these health problems or makes them disappear altogether.

You may not have to slim down very much to experience these wonderful health improvements. After losing as little as 10 or 20 pounds, many black people find that their blood pressure falls, their blood-sugar profile improves (if they have diabetes), and their joint pain starts to diminish. And best of all, they feel like a new person.

At the same time, it's important not to turn concern for weight into an unhealthy obsession. Someone once said, "A woman can never be too rich or too thin." Well, women (men, too) *can* be too thin. Undernourishment can cause bone thinning, slow healing, disruption of your hormones, and a shorter lifespan, not to mention placing you at risk for an eating disorder. And studies say it's people who starve themselves, drink themselves, or smoke themselves into pencil thinness who suffer these health risks, not people who are just naturally thin due to genetics. So as black folks who in a moment of weakness might be tempted to aim extra hard for the supermodel look because we're a bit heavier than the American average, we can't afford to go overboard on the weight-loss thing.

What's the best way for those of us struggling with a

weight problem to improve our health? How can we minimize our chances of developing health problems later in life? How does obesity affect African-Americans? Why is it so prevalent? If we or someone we love is carrying extra pounds, when should we be concerned? Why should we be concerned? For black folks who happen to be large and who want to be the happiest, the sanest, and the most peaceful people we can be, what are our most realistic options?

These questions are what this book is all about.

CHAPTER 2

What's So Bad About Being Fat?

Have you taken a close look at a box of pancake mix lately? Aunt Jemima doesn't have the same plump physique that you may remember from your childhood. In 1968, the Quaker Oats company slimmed down Aunt Jemima to bring her image more in line with modern expectations.

Aunt Jemima isn't the only corporate logo with a slimmer, trimmer look. When the *Wall Street Journal* did some checking, they discovered that Psyche, the winged goddess who's perched atop White Rock beverage labels, had been whittled down from what the company says was 140 pounds a century ago to an estimated 118 pounds today. Even the cherubic Campbell Kids were redrawn in a 1983 campaign to show the soup company's self-professed concern for well-being. When customers complained that the children had lost their innocence and looked too serious, the company reversed the facelift, returning the youngsters to their former pudginess. That prompted one nutritionist at the Good Housekeeping Institute to complain that despite medical advice against placing children on diets, "Cherubs are out and athletes are in."

Such is the state of America's fascination with thinness. We celebrate it in our advertising. We glorify it in our fashions. We pay homage to it in our restaurant menus. In pursuit of the slender body, we pump iron and take up sports, have our thighs tucked and stomachs stapled, forgo meals and skip snacks. And we dream dreams of how we would look if we could only force those hips down to a size 8 (or 14 or 22) or how handsome we'd be if we could just deflate the spare tire around our middle.

Americans aren't the only ones concerned with thinness. In Africa, where millions face the threat of having too little to eat, urban residents have begun to fashion their lifestyles after the abundance of the West. Traditional diets of whole grains and modest amounts of fat and protein are giving way to refined grains, alcohol, and sweets. The traditionally relaxed pace of life is being replaced by the stresses of deadlines and factory time clocks. And as urbanized Africans increasingly take up Western ways, they begin to mirror a Western fondness for slimness as well.

In China, where for generations peasants have struggled to coax a meager existence from unyielding soil, obesity has traditionally meant prosperity. Not anymore. Food is now plentiful in much of China, and chagrined Chinese are discovering that being overweight is no picnic. "The biggest problem is that I can't find clothes anywhere," one 290-pound, sixteen-year-old boy told the *New York Times*. In Shanghai, a high-fashion city with a distinctive Western flair, women line up for weight-loss treatments at a special ward of the Xiangshan Chinese Medical Hospital. A nurse smears their bellies with rhubarb paste, a supposed flab melter, then attaches electrodes from a Multipurpose Passive Exerciser that flash as they silently massage quivering abdomens. "It is very comfortable, like taking a sleeping pill," one patient explains to a reporter. Never mind that the treatment is a bust; when it comes to losing weight the journey is as important as the destination, even in China.

In America, chubby children are still shuffled off to weight-reduction camps and dieters of all ages latch on to whatever new gimmick promises the most painless weight loss. It's the degree of obsession that sets America apart from every other nation. The relentless drive for thinness saturates American culture, rendering fat people objects of pity, if not ridicule. In the face of this remarkable pressure to conform to a slender ideal, more and more hefty people are doing something quite radical. They're saying they like themselves just fine the way they are, thank you. What the arbiters of social acceptability feel is immaterial, these fat people say; what counts is how fat people feel about themselves.

IS FAT WHERE IT'S AT?

Flip through the pages of those new magazines for large women—publications like *Big Beautiful Women (BBW), Dimensions,* or *MODE*—and you won't find many people spilling crocodile tears over their dress sizes. What you'll find are women who love themselves and love their bodies. These are the voices of women who are quite satisfied with their weight, thank you very much, and can find no earthly reason to step on an endless diet treadmill that probably won't work anyway.

Big people haven't always felt this sense of solidarity. Some trace today's more-positive self-images of large-bodied folks back to the mid-1980s, when William "The Refrigerator" Perry walked into the Chicago Bears football camp. Perry, a gifted 300-pound defensive lineman who has since retired, proved immensely popular throughout the country but especially in Chicago, where he even inspired his own cheering squad—a passel of chunky cheerleaders called "The Refrigerettes."

By the late 1980s, fat people took their advocacy

Folks Who Feel Fat Is Fine

In 1969, William Fabrey finally got fed up with the ridicule suffered by his wife and others who are larger than average. Fabrey, who weighs 210 pounds, founded NAAFA—the National Association to Advance Fat Acceptance—a nonprofit 1,500-member group based in Sacramento, California. One of the most difficult challenges for fat people is accepting—and liking—who they are. But groups like NAAFA provide a measure of reassurance and comraderie that can build self-esteem. Witness Mary-Jane Grace-Brown, a 400-pound NAAFA member who with calm and grace has endured strangers yanking doughnuts from her shopping cart and rebuking her for overeating, and inquiries from incredulous television audiences about how she and her husband make love. The secret to her even temper, Grace-Brown says, is an inner peace. "Even at five pounds overweight, people have no self-esteem or are so diet-oriented that they are almost jealous of people who accept themselves as they are," Grace-Brown told the *Atlanta Constitution*. "They just can't seem to handle someone else being happy and fat."

For more information, contact:
NAAFA
P.O. Box 188620
Sacramento, CA 95818
(916) 558-6880, or (800) 442-1214 for membership information
Web site: www.naafa.org
E-mail: naafa@naafa.org

work a step further by demanding their constitutional rights. Citing job discrimination, 100 NAAFA members rallied in Baltimore to suggest that freedom from discrimination based on body weight should be a constitutionally protected civil right. Harry Gossett, author of *Fat Chance,* a book on discrimination against fat people, compared weight discrimination to race discrimination. Borrowing from Dr. Martin Luther King's "I Have a Dream" speech, Gossett told the crowd, "We have a similar dream: for people to be judged by their ability and not by their attraction to gravity."

Not too long thereafter, overweight employees began to file a string of court cases, challenging their employer's right to dictate hiring, promotions, and firing on the basis of weight. One of the first victories for employees came in Baltimore, when a judge ruled in 1990 that four overweight women had been unfairly denied jobs as bus drivers. The women, all of whom weighed around 200 pounds, had been turned away not because they couldn't drive and clean buses, but because the Maryland Mass Transit Administration perceived them as being incapable of doing so.

That, in a nutshell, is the prevailing attitude fat people are fighting—the instantaneous, deep-seated perception of inferiority. "We got fat, not stupid," Joyce Rue-Potter, founder of Abundantly Yours, a San Diego–based support group, told the *Los Angeles Times.* "But a lot of people equate sluggish of body, sluggish of mind."

That attitude may change as more courts rule in favor of obese employees. Hollywood may help, too, by continuing to insist, as one producer put it, that it's respectable to not fit into a pair of size 10 Calvins. In that sense, television may be helping large Americans gain a bit of self-esteem by providing positive role models.

ISN'T IT RISKY TO BE FAT?

It's not just big people who are beginning to question the conventional wisdom about obesity. Americans as a whole are becoming more accepting as well. One survey by the Chicago–based NPG group found that America's hard line against overweight people may be softening. The group discovered that the number of Americans who agreed that slender people are more attractive than fat people fell from 55 percent to 42 percent in a span of just four years.

Even doctors give some fat patients a clean bill of health. "I feel better than I've ever felt in my life," Ruby Greenwald, who is 5 feet 8 inches tall and weighs 350 pounds, told a *New York Times* reporter. "And the doctor can't find anything wrong with me—except that I'm fat." Indeed, some physicians believe the risks of obesity have been grossly exaggerated. They say people who are only 10 or 15 pounds overweight don't substantially increase their chances of developing health problems.

There's some evidence from South Africa to back this claim. Researchers there found that a group of 210 poor rural black women had very few weight-related health problems despite an obesity rate of nearly 20 percent. The women were very physically active and enjoyed a low-fat, mostly vegetarian diet of corn, brown bread, seasonal fruits and vegetables, beans, and occasional dairy products and meat. When few of the women showed high blood pressure, elevated blood cholesterol levels, or other typical markers of obesity, the researchers wondered whether they had stumbled on a phenomenon they termed "healthy obesity."

Perhaps so, but not all African obesity is benign. Other studies show that overweight Africans run a high risk of hypertension, heart disease, and other deadly complications. According to researchers at the University of Natal in South Africa, African urbanization and the adoption of Western lifestyles have sent obesity rates—and disease rates—soaring. Heart attacks, which were virtually unknown for years, account for some 12 percent of all heart-related disease among black Africans in Johannesburg. And high blood pressure is now common among urban blacks.

In the United States, too, obesity is responsible for a tremendous range of serious, life-threatening conditions and diseases. Even mild obesity—say, 20 or 30 pounds above a person's "ideal" weight—heightens the risk of health problems. Let's take a closer look at the ways that too much body fat can hurt your physical health, your emotional well-being, and even your wallet.

Physical Health

In the summer of 1987, on the way to the bathroom in his Long Island home, Walter Hudson fell and couldn't get up. When rescue workers answered the call, they were shocked to find a 1,200-pound black man sprawled on his belly.

Walter Hudson had always been heavy. As a twelve-year-old, he weighed 375 pounds. By age forty-two, his abdomen measured nine feet around. "I was addicted to food, the same way an alcoholic is addicted to liquor," he told *Parade* magazine. As Hudson grew massive, so did his health problems: headaches, backaches, arthritis, wheezing. It hurt so much to move about that Hudson spent most of his life in bed, walking as little as possible, and then with the aid of an aluminum crutch that he would hold in front of him like the third leg of a tripod.

By 1988, Hudson was convinced by his accident—it took rescue workers 4½ hours to lift him—that he needed to lose weight. What if his house had been on fire? he wondered. So he started on Dick Gregory's powdered Bahamian diet supplement and over the months proceeded to lose 600 pounds. He said he just wanted to live a normal life.

Walter Hudson never got that chance. On Christmas Eve, 1991, at the early age of forty-six, he died. The coroner said the cause of death was heart failure brought on by morbid obesity.

Walter Hudson was clearly an extreme example of what can happen when a person's weight gets out of hand. Yet the Hudson case has become a powerful symbol of the impact of body weight on millions of less heavy members of the black community.

Being fat can be an annoyance, and it can be an embarrassment. But it's much more than that. "We want the average American to know that obesity is a disease," says Dr. Jules Hirsch, who chaired an expert panel commissioned by the National Institutes of Health (NIH) to evaluate the risks of being fat. "And it carries with it a risk for increased mortality [death]." It was the most sobering and broad-reaching pronouncement on the subject to date; one observer likened it to the Surgeon General's pivotal 1964 warning about smoking.

The NIH report was based, among other things, on

studies that tracked the health of large groups of people for many years. One such study found that the average fat person in their thirties will develop a life-threatening medical condition in about eight years for men, and fourteen years for women. The implications were enormous. "We're committing national suicide," one researcher said bluntly. Black Americans typically have more preexisting health problems—diabetes, hypertension, heart disease—than do whites, which make our chances of developing weight-related life-threatening problems even greater. Black physicians know this, and their message to black Americans is loud and clear. "Being normal weight or thin is not good just for aesthetic reasons," Dr. Tazewell Banks, professor of medicine at Howard University, told *Ebony*. "It adds five to fifteen years to a person's life."

While obesity is often hazardous, not all body fat is alike. About 25 percent of all overweight people—mostly men, but some women—have round stomachs that give them the profile of an apple. Another 25 percent—mostly women, but some men—have fatty buttocks and thighs that make them resemble a pear. (The remaining 50 percent have body shapes that lie in between.) If you're shaped like an apple, you run a much higher risk of developing a number of fat-related conditions, including heart disease, hypertension, diabetes, stroke, and even breast cancer in women.

Why does fat location make such a big difference? Researchers aren't sure. They do know that belly fat enters the bloodstream easier than hip fat does. Belly fat disturbs the body's cholesterol equilibrium, sending unhealthy LDL (low-density lipoprotein) cholesterol into a person's arteries. That may be a reason that "apple" physiques suffer higher rates of heart dis-

Are You an Apple or a Pear?

It's easy to figure your body type. Measure your waist at its narrowest point, then measure your hips at their widest point. Then divide the waist measurement by the hip measurement. If you're a man, consider yourself a pear if the number you get is below .80 and an apple if the number is above .95. Women are pears if their number is below .75 and apples if the number is above .85.

For example, let's say your narrowest waist measurement is 40 inches, and your widest hip measurement is 60 inches. Dividing the hips by the waist means 40 divided by 60, or .66. For both women and men, that qualifies as a pear shape.

ease. Researchers also know that the cells inside apple-shaped bodies don't seem to react normally to insulin, the hormone that allows the body to use glucose for food. That could be why apples face a high risk of diabetes.

One thing that *is* clear is why obese men and women tend to have different body shapes. It's all about evolution. Since prehistoric times, males have taken charge of foraging and hunting, two tasks that frequently took men on expeditions ranging far from reliable food supplies. Men who could store excess food (in the form of fat) in their abdomens had an important advantage over men who couldn't, because their extra fat functioned like a camel's hump, carrying them through lean times when food wasn't available. Unlike hip and buttocks fat, abdominal fat is easily converted to energy, so that the "hump" was always there, ready to provide much-needed calories at a moment's notice.

Women, on the other hand, are the only humans capable of childbearing. Their extra fat cushions and protects their reproductive organs from injury. Thigh and hip fat is also much more difficult to lose (a fact discovered by many dieters). The one exception is during pregnancy and nursing, when thigh and hip fat becomes readily available, if needed, to help supply mother and child with crucial calories. Here again, the reason is survival. Thousands of years ago women were no more assured of a steady food supply than men were. So their bodies developed a way to hold on to extra calories and store them for childbearing, the one act whose success is vital to the continuation of the species.

The good news here is that whether you're an apple or a pear or somewhere in between, your health risks can decrease, sometimes dramatically, when you adopt a healthful lifestyle. Let's examine some of the most troublesome physical problems linked with obesity, and how those problems can be eased once you lose weight. Bear in mind that not everyone who is overweight suffers from the conditions listed below. Though carrying a great deal of weight heightens the risk of these health problems, some fat people are perfectly healthy.

Obesity and Hypertension If you're black, you have an increased risk of high blood pressure, the bane of the black community. On the average, African-Americans have nearly a 33 percent greater chance of having hypertension than whites do, and when we get it, it's more severe.

But if you're black and overweight, your chances of having or developing high blood pressure are even greater. Federal studies of some 20,000 adults—some 5,000 of them African-Americans—showed that obese middle-aged blacks are 20 percent more likely than are average-weight blacks in the same age group to have high blood pressure. Even in young black adults —persons we often assume are relatively immune from life-threatening disease—obesity increases the risk of hypertension by as much as 260 percent.

What's the connection between body weight and hypertension? The leading theory points to the kidneys. Human kidneys are miniature filtration factories. Every 24 hours, all of the blood in the body filters through the kidneys an average of 500 to 600 times. This remarkable feat is accomplished with the help of long filtering tubes called *nephrons.* Once blood enters a kidney, waste products such as water, sodium (salt), and ammonia are pushed from the bloodstream into the nephrons, where the liquid waste gradually becomes concentrated. What emerges at the end of this filtration process is urine.

The average kidney contains around 1 million nephrons. But some overweight people have fewer than that. This nephron deficit sets off a whole chain reaction. Fewer nephrons means that less sodium gets filtered from the bloodstream. And when that happens, we retain fluid. That's because the body can tolerate sodium only in small amounts, so we need water to dilute the sodium down to a safe level. The extra water that we retain is great for dilution, but it fills our arteries with excess fluid. And that contributes to high blood pressure.

While many overweight people have high blood pressure, not all do. The reason may be that not every fat person has too few nephrons. If the kidneys are normal, they may be able to handle their filtering responsibilities without a sodium buildup. But if they have a nephron deficit, each additional pound of body weight means that more and more blood must circulate through weary, overtaxed nephrons. The heavier a person's body weight, the less efficiently their kidneys can filter out sodium, and the greater the risk of hypertension.

You've undoubtedly heard black folks voice more and more concern for their "pressure" as they grow older. There's a medical basis for that: While some of us manage to have normal blood pressure throughout our lives, blood pressure typically increases with age. As people grow older, their once-flexible arteries become less elastic and more rigid. This reduces the arteries' ability to momentarily bulge to accommodate each pulse of blood from the heart. Without this valuable shock absorber, pressure from each heartbeat is contained within a stiffened blood vessel instead of being safely dampened. As a result, pressure builds up inside the artery—pressure that can eventually lead to a stroke or heart disease.

But there's a twist. While blood pressure typically increases as a person grows older, so does body weight. And the two may be closely related. "In populations where there is not an age-related body weight increase, an elevation of blood pressure with age is not apparent," writes Dr. F. X. Pi-Sunyer, professor of medicine at New York's St. Luke's/Roosevelt Hospital Center. So in addition to hypertension medication and regular exercise, weight control can be an important way to prevent hypertension, especially (but not exclusively) in older persons.

In fact, for every 25 pounds that you lose, your blood pressure can fall an average of 21 (systolic) and 13 (diastolic) points, respectively. Doctors say you can use these numbers to estimate how much you can lower your blood pressure by reducing your weight. (See box below.)

One Way to Lower Your Blood Pressure: Lose Weight

Let's say you weigh 225 pounds and your doctor warns you that you have high blood pressure. The first thing to do is ask what the actual blood pressure numbers are. We'll assume the doctor says 165/100, which corresponds to moderate hypertension.

The rule of thumb is that for every 25 pounds of weight that you lose, your blood pressure falls an average of 21 systolic and 13 diastolic points. That means by slimming down from 225 to 200 pounds, you could reduce your blood pressure from 165/100 to 144/87. In one fell swoop, you will have brought your hypertension from the moderate range to the mild range.

Another 25 pounds of weight loss could lower your blood pressure to around 123/74, which is in the normal range. Weight reduction can be a tremendous tool in the fight for good health.

Obesity and Heart Disease Your heart is a single organ, but it's really made of four separate chambers. Each chamber works in concert with the others so that every heartbeat is a smooth, coordinated partnership.

Now imagine one of those chambers growing in size. The larger it gets, the less it fits with the other three normal-size chambers, and the more difficult it is for the heart to pump in unison. In time, what started as a well-oiled, finely tuned pump becomes uncoordinated and lopsided, like a washing machine tossing around an unbalanced load. Eventually, the heart does what a stressed-out washing machine does: it stops.

That's just one of the ways that obesity can lead to heart disease. When you gain weight, your body manufactures more blood to carry oxygen and other nutrients to the newly added fat tissue. With more blood to pump, the heart is forced to take on a larger workload. As you gain more and more pounds, the *left ventricle,* the heart chamber most responsible for ejecting blood from the heart and pushing it through thousands of blood vessels throughout the body, eventually becomes overdeveloped and enlarged, causing a condition called *left ventricular hypertrophy.* In time, the left ventricle fails, the heart shuts down, and the person suffers what we know as a heart attack.

Heart disease is the number one killer of Americans. It claimed almost 1 million lives in 1995—more than the next seven leading causes of death combined—and it's a disease that strikes the black community with a vengeance. Black men die from heart disease at a rate 49 percent higher than for white men, and the death rate for black women is a sky-high 67 percent higher than for white women.

Why such a big difference in black and white fatality rates? The major reason is that African-Americans have more conditions that place us at risk for heart disease. These so-called *risk factors* are not only more prevalent in our community, but also more severe.

Hypertension is a prime example. It runs rampant in the black community, although more and more African-Americans are learning to control the condition through medication, diet, and exercise. Hypertension leads to heart disease because high blood pressure strains the heart. High blood pressure also damages the lining of the blood vessels, creating a buildup of fatty deposits that can eventually block an artery, causing a stroke (if the obstruction blocks the blood flow to the brain) or a heart attack (if it lodges in the arteries that feed the heart).

Another risk factor for heart disease is too much

cholesterol and other fatty sludge in the bloodstream. You've no doubt heard of the damage these infamous artery cloggers can cause.

And let's not forget cigarette smoking, another risk factor for heart disease. African-Americans smoke fewer cigarettes than whites do, but we tend to smoke brands that have higher amounts of cancer-causing tar, according to the U.S. Department of Human Services Office on Smoking and Health.

Both hypertension and bloodstream fats, the two most important risk factors for heart disease, are aggravated by excess body weight.

In fact, National Institutes of Health researchers

Why Do Smokers Have So Much Heart Disease?

For years, doctors have known that cigarette smoke is nearly as hard on our hearts as it is on our lungs. The nicotine in smoke makes the heart race, increases blood pressure, and sends fats pouring into the bloodstream.

But at Boston's Brigham and Women's Hospital, researchers think they've uncovered another reason that cigarettes hurt the heart. It's all about "spare tires." When smokers gain weight, they're slightly more likely than nonsmokers to add the extra pounds around their middles. Since belly fat is more likely to cause heart disease than is hip fat, this may be one reason why cigarette smokers have more heart problems.

have estimated that obesity is responsible for up to one-third of the hypertension in the black community, and one-tenth of the high cholesterol.

Researchers from Harvard, furthermore, found that fully 40 percent of the heart attacks and heart disease in clinically overweight women, and 70 percent of the heart disease in clinically obese women, could be traced to the women's weight—a finding believed applicable to men as well. This surprising discovery, based on a study of over 100,000 nurses, showed that weight-related heart problems were much more serious than previously believed. Researchers now believe that one of the reasons that black women die more often than white women do from heart disease (as well as from stroke and hypertension) is that black women weigh more. That could hold true for black men as well. Imagine how many of our relatives and friends and neighbors might live longer, fuller, happier, more productive lives if we could only slow the toll of weight-related heart disease.

It *can* be done, and it's *being* done across the country by black Americans who are concerned about their own health and about the welfare of their loved ones. Many of us are keeping closer tabs on our diet, particularly the greasy favorites—you know the ones—that increase our blood cholesterol levels, and the salty standbys that contribute to high blood pressure. And we're exercising—jogging and swimming, leaping into aerobics and jazzercise classes, thwacking racketballs and tennis balls.

Watching what we eat and getting regular exercise are not only great ways to put a lid on the biggest risk factors for heart disease (hypertension and blood fats). They're also the safest and most effective way to lose weight. We'll explore how to construct a sensible eating and exercise program in Chapters 5 and 6.

Obesity and Diabetes From the northernmost Eskimos to the South African Bantus, from East to West and back again, the human race is a portrait of staggering biological diversity. We differ from each other in skin tone, body build, hair texture, eye color, and a hundred other ways.

But in every culture you'll find one constant: The more people weigh, the more likely they are to have diabetes. Whether it's Finland or Florida, New Zealand or New York, obesity and diabetes are two peas in a pod. Here in America, where black people of all ages have a greater risk of (1) developing diabetes, (2) having more severe complications, and (3) dying from the disease than do whites, up to half of all cases of diabetes in the black community are thought to stem from excess body weight. In fact, many researchers consider obesity a "prediabetic" state.

To understand why, you need to know a little about a powerful hormone called *insulin.* After we eat a meal, the juices in our digestive tract break down the food into its simplest components. Much of it ends up as *glucose,* a sugar that the body uses for fuel. Every working cell relies on glucose for the energy it needs to function. But the glucose we get from food winds up in the bloodstream, far away from the individual brain, muscle, and other cells that desperately need it. Somehow the glucose must find its way to its ultimate destination—these billions of living cells from head to foot.

How does the body pull off such a logistical coup? With insulin. Insulin is a glucose transporter. In healthy people, it latches onto glucose in the bloodstream and neatly delivers it throughout the body. Think of insulin as a team of expert mail carriers delivering life-giving packages to far-flung destinations.

Now imagine those mail carriers on strike. Or struggling against the worst blizzard imaginable. With no distribution system, the packages start to pile up at the source. And the more the mail carriers are unavailable, the more the entire system suffers.

That, in a nutshell, is diabetes. Diabetics have one

of two problems: either their bodies produce too little insulin (the glucose carrier), or the body produces plenty of insulin but certain factors don't allow the hormone to do its job. Either way, glucose accumulates in the bloodstream (which is why diabetics have high blood sugar). Over the years, this disturbance in glucose metabolism can eventually snowball into telltale signs that are all too familiar in the black community: skin sores that won't heal, vision problems that slowly worsen, kidney disease (frequently necessitating costly dialysis), hardening of the arteries (atherosclerosis), and often amputation and premature death.

How does body weight factor into all of this? As it turns out, large bodies aren't very responsive to insulin. The pancreas, an insulin-producing gland tucked behind the stomach, tries to produce more of the hormone to try to compensate, but it eventually fails to keep up with the stream of glucose entering into the bloodstream. (This is why diabetics must sometimes take insulin—to make up for the insulin the pancreas can't produce.) The end result of this sugar overload is diabetes.

Being fat doesn't invariably cause diabetes, but it triples your risk of developing the disease. Other risk factors include belly fat—the "apple" physique—and a family history of diabetes. These are all important considerations for African-Americans, given how widespread diabetes is in our community.

Fortunately, diabetes can be controlled and even reversed. According to the Center for Science in the Public Interest, a Washington, D.C.–based nutrition group, a healthful diet—one low in fat and high in carbohydrates and fiber—may help diabetics as much as insulin does. Exercise helps control diabetes, too.

And let's not forget losing weight, which can make an obese person once again sensitive to insulin, thus restoring the glucose transport system to full and healthy efficiency.

Obesity and Cancer If someone were to ask you to name something that causes cancer, you might mention cigarettes or too much sun. But did you know that body weight is linked with cancer, too? When the American Cancer Society followed over 700,000 adults for thirteen years, the risk of cancer was related to people's body weight. Persons who weighed over 40 percent of their "ideal" weight had a higher death rate compared to those who weighed less. Obese people as a whole had a higher risk of colon and rectal cancer. Overweight women developed cancer of certain of their reproductive organs (uterus, ovaries, endometrium, cervix, and breast), along with the gallbladder. Obese men developed more cancer of the prostate.

Speculation is that reproductive-organ cancers—which account for half of all cancers in women—may be tied to estrogen, the female hormone. Fatty tissue produces a steady stream of estrogen, and being fat also causes the body to manufacture additional estrogen from a related hormone. Researchers think this estrogen overload causes cancer by interfering with reproductive-organ tissues, which are sensitive to the hormone.

Breast cancer is another disease that seems to be tied to a person's weight. One 1997 Yale University study found that black women who are severely obese tend to have more advanced—and less treatable—breast cancer than do whites. Cancer researchers know that racial differences often come about because black folks generally have lower incomes than whites, and have less access to screening and treatment. But in this case, the racial differences persisted even after taking into account socioeconomic status and access to health care. So what's going on here? The answers may lie, once again, with hormones: Women who are severely overweight have more estrogen in their bodies. "If a tumor is growing rapidly," one researcher told the *Washington Post,* "the hypothesis is that the extra load of estrogen may promote more rapid growth." The researchers also found a link between occupational status and breast cancer, with women who hold lower-status jobs being more likely to have more advanced breast cancer.

Colorectal cancers, on the other hand, may stem from bile, a greenish liquid that's produced in the liver to help us digest fats. Bile acts as a detergent to break up fat into small droplets that the body can absorb. When we eat high-fat diets, our livers manufacture lots of bile, which mixes with the food during digestion and eventually makes its way into the large intestine. Scientists suspect that excess bile salts, one of the components of bile, may promote cancer in the lower digestive tract. That might explain why fat people—whose diets may be particularly high in fats and cholesterol—are prone to these cancers.

Obesity and Arthritis Many of the 206 bones in the body move against each other, and those that do are typically protected with a smooth layer of cartilage. The cartilage acts as a shock absorber and a cushion, allowing knees to flex and elbows to bend without direct, bone-to-bone contact. Excess body weight can subject this cartilage to inordinate wear and tear. The task of supporting more weight than the body may have been built for can eventually make normally smooth cartilage rough and cracked. Over time, a joint can lose much of its cushioning, resulting in a painful and sometimes disabling condition known as *osteoarthritis*—the most common form of arthritis. In fact, if you're obese, you have a 2 to 1 risk of developing osteoarthritis if you're a man, and a 3 to 1 risk if you're a woman.

Obesity doesn't cause arthritis, but it does worsen it. Arthritis (especially of the knees, hips, or spine) is a common complaint in fat people. Fortunately, the pain and disability from weight-related arthritis can be eased with weight reduction.

(By the way, if you know anyone who has put off exercising because they say they're afraid of developing arthritis, tell them to start looking for their sweatpants—

Does Affluence Protect Blacks from the Health Effects of Obesity?

It's been said that poverty lies at the root of many problems that confront the African-American community. That's clearly true with many health problems. Poverty often means difficult access to health facilities, inadequate or nonexistent health insurance, and inferior care from overcrowded, understaffed public hospitals and clinics. And as we've seen, obesity—and presumably its many side effects—is more pronounced among poor black women than among more affluent ones.

But does money help black Americans escape the health risks of being fat? The Centers for Disease Control and Prevention (CDC) once studied that question in a group of 8,800 adults—one-tenth of them black—from throughout the country who were followed for ten years. CDC looked at six risk factors, four of which (hypertension, blood cholesterol level, diabetes, and body-mass index) are associated with obesity.

> The scientists discovered that 38 percent of the so-called excess deaths in black adults were attributable to family income. So the higher your income, the more you can avoid a substantial proportion — up to 38 percent — of the health risk associated with being African-American. But the flip side of the 38 percent figure means that 62 percent of the excess deaths had nothing to do with income. CDC thinks this figure could encompass items like exercise, which is known to keep people healthy regardless of their income.

there's no connection. Stanford University researchers have found that even marathon runners don't have an increased chance of getting arthritis in their knees, ankles, or hips. "The risk of getting arthritis can no longer be an excuse for all those people lying on the couch on Sunday afternoon," one researcher told the *Boston Globe.*)

Obesity and Birth Defects We don't often think about obesity harming anyone but the person who's carrying those extra pounds. But obese women who become pregnant double their chance of giving birth to a baby with a serious neural-tube defect, such as spina bifida (incomplete closure of the spinal column) or anencephaly (missing brain). In one study, completed in 1996 at Boston University, women who weighed 176 to 195 pounds were about twice as likely to have a child with a neural-tube defect as women who weighed 110 to 130 pounds. In a second study, the same risk was associated with women with a body-mass index higher than 29. There's some evidence that actual body weight isn't the only issue; some researchers say that if your weight is appropriate for your height, you're in the clear. Otherwise, no one really understands why obesity and birth defects are linked. Scientists speculate the extra body fat may cause an abnormality in the mother's metabolism, but they're not sure.

Obesity and Disability in the Elderly When black folks age, they share at least one attribute with whites: They often eat less. Some people gradually lose their taste for food, a process hastened by the slow deterioration of the taste buds and a diminished level of physical activity, which helps quell a person's appetite by slowing his or her metabolism. Some people's stomachs shrink when they age, which means that they feel full after eating smaller meals than when they were younger. Whatever the reason, African-Americans often weigh less in their sixties, seventies, and eighties than they did in their thirties, forties, and fifties.

If an older person happens to be heavy, their weight might understandably cause some amount of disability. (Arthritis is a good example of a debilitating weight-related disease that limits a person's activities.) But it may surprise you to know that a mere history of obesity can lead to disability later in life—even if an elder isn't presently fat. In one study, researchers at the University of South Carolina Department of Biometry quizzed over 1,000 men and women, one-third of them black, to understand why people grow disabled in older age. The participants, whose average age was around seventy, were asked how easily they could perform a number of everyday tasks (dressing, eating, walking across a room, writing, standing in one place for more than fifteen minutes, and so forth). As it turned out, African-Americans had significantly more disability than did whites. Black women had the highest prevalence of disability: 56 percent—over half—could not perform the tasks in question. (The comparable figure for white women was 43 percent.) Among black men, 39 percent were disabled, compared to 26 percent for white males. Interestingly, the researchers posed the same questions to a group of affluent black men who were only slightly younger (average age: sixty-four years) than the others. These black men reported a disability level of barely 22 percent—the lowest of any group studied.

When the researchers examined the factors that predispose older persons for disability, they found that age, high blood pressure, and the presence of heart disease were reliable predictors, especially in black men. But for black women, a history of obesity was a strong predictor of later disability. You can see why experts say that while losing excess weight is a good idea at any age, it's even better to try to stay a healthy size to begin with.

Emotional Health

No panel of scientific experts has ever studied the human side of obesity—the emotional distress, the embarrassment of public humiliation, the continual struggle of overweight people forced to cope with a world geared to the slender. No expert has to proclaim what fat people already know—that life for the obese is a singular experience. Marilyn Lewis, a black woman and native of Baltimore, spoke candidly to *Ebony* magazine about her everyday challenges—squeezing behind the steering wheel of a car, shopping for a size 60 dress, freezing in winter because she can't find close-toed shoes wide enough to accommodate her feet. "Unless you have ever been morbidly obese, it is impossible to comprehend how difficult it is for a fat person to live in a world tailored for the thin." As one man, hospitalized for serious complications he suffered after stomach surgery reduced his weight from 400 to 200 pounds, told the *Washington Post,* "Even as I lie here feeling I could die, there is no question that I would go through the operations again. They changed my life in ways that a normal-weight person can never begin to imagine."

Many of these frustrations become apparent as soon as large people set foot in public. Most public facilities are designed to accommodate people half the size of many African-Americans. Going to a restaurant that doesn't have wide armless chairs is futile, and trying to squeeze into a booth is next to impossible. Fat people give thanks for movie rentals, because they can't fit into theater seats. On airplanes, after having to request an extended seat belt, they squish their seatmates, who aren't always sympathetic. "People really get upset about this and they're not the least bit shy about complaining," one travel publisher told the *Wall Street Journal.*

People receive unmistakable cultural messages about body weight at an early age. When schoolchildren as young as five years old are asked to choose the least likable child among drawings of youngsters with various physical characteristics, including missing hands and disfigured faces, they invariably pick the drawing of the fat child. Researchers find the same tendency among adults and, sadly, among fat people as well.

According to a study at the Harvard School of Public Health, overweight high school graduates are less likely than others to be accepted at top colleges, even when they have the same credentials as average-weight students. If they manage to get into college, they still face an uphill road. Dr. Esther Rothblum, a University of Vermont psychologist who studies weight discrimination, tells of a college student whose professor stopped in midlecture to ask, "When are you going to lose weight? You're too fat." Sharon Russell, a 5-foot-6-inch, 300-pound nursing student at Rhode Island's Salve Regina University, says that her instructors harassed her for months about her weight. They used her to demonstrate how to give a fat person an injection, and how to make a bed for a fat person. "Sharon, lie down," the instructor called out. After school officials pressured her into signing a contract to attend Weight Watchers meetings and to lose two pounds a week, Russell sued the college. (The case went to the U.S. Supreme Court, which ruled in favor of the university, partly because Russell admitted that her weight was caused by overeating.)

Colleges aren't the only institutions concerned about their image, and how fat people might tarnish it. Employers often consider obese employees about as welcome as an IRS audit. It's one thing to be concerned about a job applicant's physical abilities, particularly when public safety is at risk; police and fire departments have well-established weight guidelines that few people question. But discrimination experts say that fat people are barred from workplaces even when their weight has nothing to do with job performance. Research by University of Pennsylvania psychiatrist Dr. Albert Stunkard shows that employers are more likely to assume that obese job applicants are poorer workers who take advantage of company sick-leave policies by feigning sickness. Some job-placement specialists estimate that it takes overweight people an average of five weeks longer than average-weight applicants to get a job. That's understandable when you consider that 44 percent of employers in one survey admitted their refusal to hire fat women under certain circumstances, and an additional 16 percent refused to hire fat women entirely. (Women are often held to higher standards of personal appearance in the workplace than are men.) That speaks highly of the overweight black women who have jobs.

Some physicians discriminate against fat people. As one psychiatrist admitted in a medical journal article, "Most physicians regard obesity as a sin and treat fat patients with disdain befitting a moral leper." When asked in a national survey, the majority of seventy-seven doctors admitted that they considered their obese patients ugly and weak-willed—an attitude that one physician speculated stems from the opinion that fat people are self-indulgent and therefore deserve retribution. That attitude prompted the following dry comment from two colleagues: "There is no evidence that retribution is of benefit to obese patients." But retribution is what many fat people—especially black women—get. "Many doctors either assume that black women are supposed to be fat, or that they never have eating disorders," says sociologist Dr. Becky Wangsguard Thompson, a specialist on eating disorders, who found that none of the women of color in her research had visited doctors because they were pessimistic that such a move would help.

CONCLUSION

In life and in death, fat people hoe no easy row. That's certainly true for hefty African-Americans, who face a double (or with women, a triple) burden. Each year brings more medical evidence of the dangers that obesity poses to our physical health. Because of our family histories of diabetes, hypertension, and other serious disease, we as African-American people are at special risk of dying before our time.

And the stigma of obesity can pose a serious threat to emotional health. Old beliefs die hard, no matter how outmoded they may be. Like the fight for racial equality, it's taking lots of hard work to begin to open the doors of access and equal opportunity for this minority whose weight makes discrimination not only easy but often legally and socially sanctioned. The history of social movements in this country shows that the spirited efforts of a committed minority can move mountains; the "weight liberation" movement will continue to unfold in the new millennium.

But let's put aside for a moment the conditions that make obesity a challenge. Sometimes we focus so hard on trying to understand the health effects of obesity or the social consequences of body weight that we lose sight of another important issue that's in some ways even more fundamental: What makes people obese to begin with?

CHAPTER 3

What Makes People Obese?

We know what makes our beautiful skin brown: our genes. And we know what keeps our muscles toned: our lifestyle. But what makes people fat?

The popular answer is simple: Fat people eat too much. Everyone knows that your body weight depends on the number of calories you eat and the number that you burn up. People who eat less than they burn lose weight. Those who eat more gain weight.

The theory boils down body weight to a balancing act. Fat people take in so much food that they tip the scales beyond their bodies' ability to get rid of the extra calories and the weight starts to pile on. It doesn't help to live in a country whose principal sign of civilization is the fast-food franchise. Food in America is characterized by at least five things: It's got variety, taste appeal, lots of fat, plenty of sugar, and it's cheap enough that most people can afford at least something to eat. When you add to that the reality that we as a nation are notoriously sedentary, having long ago given up walking for driving and shovels for bulldozers, you end up with a dangerous combination indeed: too much food and too little exercise. No wonder so many Americans are fat. Or so the theory goes.

But what about the exceptions? Why can two people eat the same amount of the same food, experience similar levels of activity and exercise, and yet gain different amounts of weight? Or even better, have weight changes in the opposite direction—one person gaining weight and the other losing it? Why are entire population groups (African-American women, for example) heavier on average than others? Do black women simply eat more and exercise less, or is there more than meets the eye?

As it turns out, there's a lot more. For one thing, body weight follows distinct patterns. Obesity and poverty often go hand in hand, as does obesity with advancing age, as we've seen. What's more, starting around puberty, women have more body fat than men do and they tend to gain more weight throughout adulthood.

Education can play a role here as well, and in a way that may surprise you. Black men with some college background, for example, are actually fatter than those who never finished high school. That's according to a recent NIH study of 5,000 young adults, which also found no association between education and obesity for black women or white men, and a negative association—meaning more education corresponded to less fatness—for white women.

And finally, obesity tends to run in families. If both of your parents were fat, you have an 80 percent chance of being fat yourself. If only one was fat, you have a 40 percent chance of being fat. If neither was fat, your chance is only 18 percent. There's also a tendency for troubled families to produce overweight children. Children are powerless to resolve marital tensions, the stresses of unemployment, the effects of drug abuse, and other serious problems, and they often turn to food for comfort.

So we know that body weight follows clear patterns. Income, age, gender, location, education, family—they all play a role. But on the other hand, none of these factors is the complete story either. In fact, we don't know the complete story yet. When it comes to understanding why people are fat, science has more speculation than answers. Dr. Phillip Gorden, director of the National Institute of Diabetes, Digestive, and Kidney Disorders, calls the whole area of obesity research "a morass with a lot of discussion and little information."

What we do know, however, is that beneath the demographic trends lie some tantalizing clues. Researchers look at the origins of obesity from two angles—biological and environmental. Both are helpful in understanding the root causes of excess body weight.

BIOLOGICAL REASONS FOR OBESITY

If you've ever felt out of control with food, if your entire being has ever fixated on a mouth-watering food fantasy, you'll probably take some comfort in the words of obesity expert Dr. Jules Hirsch: "We are absolutely convinced that when a person says he can't control his eating, there is a biological basis for it."

Dr. Hirsch is one of a growing number of researchers who think there are unmistakable biological differences between fat people and average-size people—differences that mean a person's weight may be largely beyond their control. If you've ever heard someone blame their weight on "glands" or "big bones," the research emerging from hospitals and university studies supports these sorts of built-in differences in body chemistry. These findings are important, given how our culture usually places the blame for obesity squarely on the behavior or personality characteristics of the person who's overweight.

The biological theories may also help explain a puzzling paradox: In a nation blanketed by regular reports about the value of good food and regular exercise, most Americans aren't doing very much to improve their health. Our nation is just as fat as we were twenty years ago, when the federal government first started to warn us to take better care of our bodies. True, some have taken up lower-calorie "lite" foods and taken on fitness routines. But most of us "appear to have sat around watching the tube and eating Big Macs and Ding Dongs," in the words of *Washington Post* writer William Booth. These new biological theories help explain why many of us who have at least tried to pry ourselves off the couch and away from junk food still haven't been able to lose much weight.

Let's take a closer look at seven leading clues that suggest obesity is a biological phenomenon. Bear in mind that more than one of the following theories may be correct. Just as there are many theories behind why people become obese, there may be many kinds of obesity.

Theory 1: Slow Metabolism

Not too long ago, ninety-five Pima Indians began periodically visiting a small room in Phoenix, Arizona, in 24-hour shifts. They were taking part in a unique body-weight study sponsored by NIH. Doctors had long known that obesity is rampant among the Pima, up to 85 percent of whom are fat by the time they reach their early twenties. Now NIH scientists wanted to know why.

The special sealed room allowed researchers to measure precisely how many calories were burned by their subjects, who weighed an average of 210 pounds. At the end of two years. the scientists announced a remarkable discovery. The Pimas who had gained the most weight had burned 80 fewer calories a day than the normal rate for their size. It may not sound like much—80 calories is the equivalent of a handful of saltine crackers. But over a two-year period, those 80 calories translate to 18 extra pounds of body fat. The connection between metabolism (the process that turns food into energy) and body weight was starting to take shape.

Meanwhile across the Atlantic, scientists were comparing infants born to fat women with those born to thin women. The children, each three months old, were studied to measure their metabolic rate over a seven-day period. By the time the babies celebrated their first birthday, those who burned the fewest calories were fat. The babies with higher metabolisms weren't.

What's more, unlike the Pima study where food intake wasn't measured, the infant study kept track of everything the mothers fed their children. And the infants who gained weight were fed no more than those who didn't.

Taken together, these two landmark studies provided the first concrete evidence that obesity is indeed tied to a person's metabolism. "Obese people are born with a handicap," announced Dr. Hirsch. They have to learn to live with it and correct for it, he said, just like people who have other handicaps.

A third piece of the puzzle came in 1997 when researchers announced that black women burn calories more slowly than white women. The news came after scientists at the University of Pennsylvania Weight and Eating Disorders Program tested the resting metabolism of a group of women who weighed an average of 224 pounds. White women in the group burned an average of 1,731 calories when they had no activity at all. But black women burned 1,638 calories—nearly 100 calories less. It was the first clue to why black women may have a harder time losing weight, and tend to be heavier, than white women. The study doesn't mean black women are destined to be fat. "They may just have to work harder" to lose weight, program director Gary Foster told *USA Today*.

These studies support what some overweight people have been claiming for years—that they eat no more, and maybe even less, than skinny people do. Earlier government surveys had found that when people were asked to recall what they had eaten in the previous 24 hours, fat people reported consuming fewer calories than did average-weight people. Other studies in which people were asked to maintain food diaries found the same results. Still there were skeptics who felt that fat people might have forgotten or been embarrassed to tell researchers all that they ate. The Pima study, the English study, and the University of Pennsylvania study all support the idea that some people can eat less than others and still put on the pounds.

Theory 2: Sluggish Nervous System

You probably know that your nervous system lets you do things. The nerves control the many muscles that allow you to sniff, smile, squeeze, and speak.

There's a second part of the nervous system, however. And although we're rarely conscious of it, it keeps us alive. The *autonomic nervous system* controls how fast our heart beats, how quickly our food is digested, and how rapidly we excrete waste. This important nerve network consists of two equivalent and opposite halves (Figure 1). One half, the *sympathetic nervous system,* generally stimulates organs and cells. It's what comes to the rescue in emergencies by speeding up our hearts, opening our airways so we get plenty of oxygen, and inhibiting digestion so we can use precious energy for more important tasks at hand. Its partner, the *parasympathetic nervous system,* slows things down after a crisis so that we don't race off into the sunset.

What in heaven's name does this have to do with body weight? Well, animals whose autonomic nervous systems are impaired wind up gaining weight. Scientists know that animals who have decreased sympathetic activity or increased parasympathetic activity eventually become fat. But not until 1988 did anyone think to measure these two functions in people.

It happened in Kentucky, where researchers at the University of Louisville Medical School and the Louisville Veterans Administration Medical Center recruited fifty-six healthy men, all but one of them white, in their late twenties and early thirties. Each man's autonomic nervous system was assessed by measuring heart rate, the presence of adrenalinlike

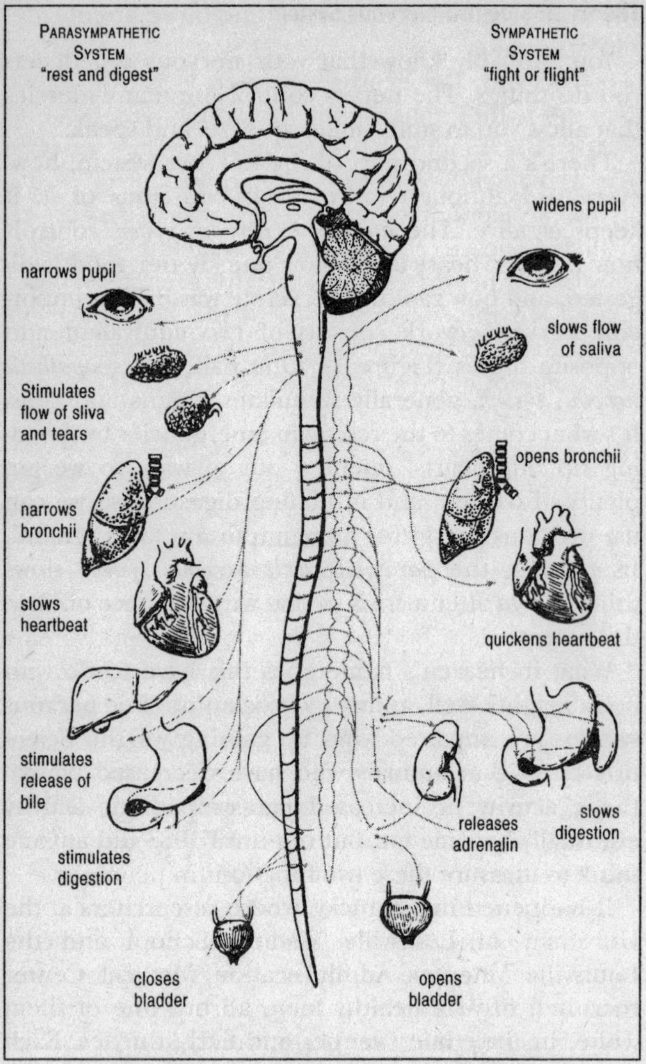

Figure 1. The sympathetic and parasympathetic nervous systems—two factors in weight control.

hormones called epinephrine and norepinephrine, and other tests.

In the end, the heavier the men were, the more depressed their autonomic nervous systems were. Sympathetic functions (which normally serve as stimulants) had slowed down—the equivalent of easing off the accelerator of a speeding car. That could explain why heavier people weigh what they do; their sympathetic nervous systems have for some reason lost steam, and the system that helps the body burn off calories is operating below par, like a furnace that's warm but not hot.

Theory 3: Obesity Genes

Is body weight inherited? More and more researchers are beginning to think so. For instance, scientists can just about predict whether a child will grow up overweight. Just look at the parents, they say. For children under age ten, having overweight parents doubles the child's chances of being a heavy adult, according to a 1997 study at Boston's New England Medical Center. In fact, the parents' size is a stronger predictor of the child's adult body size than is the child's own weight. This parental influence seems to gradually diminish, so that by adolescence the child's weight is the more important predictor.

One implication: If your toddler is pudgy and you and your spouse aren't, you shouldn't be overly concerned that the little one is going to grow up to be too heavy. (Even if all three of you are overweight, "it doesn't mean putting the kid on a diet," says Dr. Robert C. Whitaker, of Children's Hospital in Cincinnati, a coauthor on the research. Just do your best to model the eating and activity habits you want your child to grow up with.)

More evidence about genes and body weight comes from studies with identical twins. For example, several years ago, scientists at Laval University in Quebec confined twelve sets of twins, all young adult males, to a college dormitory for 100 days. There the men enjoyed a lifestyle that some might consider idyllic: plenty of food (1,000 extra calories per day, in fact) and virtually no physical activity (to avoid different amounts of exercise by each person confusing the results).

At the end of the three-month experiment, the men gained vastly different amounts of weight. One put on 9½ pounds; another gained 30. "I was astonished to see such a wide range of response," Claude Bouchard, an exercise physiologist who conducted the study, told the *Washington Post.* "There are clearly people at risk, much more than others, to gain fat."

But that's not all. Between each set of twins, the weight gain was remarkably similar. If one twin added 11 or 27 or 16 pounds, the other gained about the same amount. Since identical twins have identical genes, the researchers decided that something in the men's genetic makeup must determine how their bodies handle excess calories.

Other studies have found that identical twins raised apart gain just as much weight as do twins raised in the same house. Here again, the implication is that a person's genes control much of their weight. Estimates vary but researchers speculate that perhaps half of all weight gain may be genetically based. The remainder has to do with our environment—the type of food we eat, how much of it we consume, how much exercise we get, and so forth.

Dr. Judith Stern, professor of nutrition and internal medicine at the University of California at Davis, has a memorable saying: Genetics loads the gun, but environment pulls the trigger. "For some people it's a hair trigger and for others it's not," she told the *Washington Post.* In other words, even if you have a genetic tendency to be overweight, your lifestyle — including your exercise and eating habits—might spell the difference between being obese or being merely overweight, or between being overweight and having normal weight.

Theory 4: Signals from Fat Cells

We all know what it's like to return home after an extended absence. The dinner table groans with our favorite dishes, the most savory homestyle cooking imaginable. And Mom watches us expectantly with one message in her smiling eyes: Eat.

Well, that's the same message overweight people get. The difference is the message says "Overeat," and it comes from the person's fat cells.

All of us, whether or not we're fat, have fat cells. The body uses these important cushions to protect internal organs and to insulate against heat loss. Under a microscope, the cells look like mounds of tiny bubbles, each one capable of holding varying degrees of fat (Figure 2). An animal with a brain disorder that causes it to grossly overeat may have fat cells that are four or five times larger than normal. Conversely, in animals that have very little food, the fat cells shrink. But under normal conditions, the fat cells of animals stay precisely the same size.

Interestingly, animals are also remarkably adept at

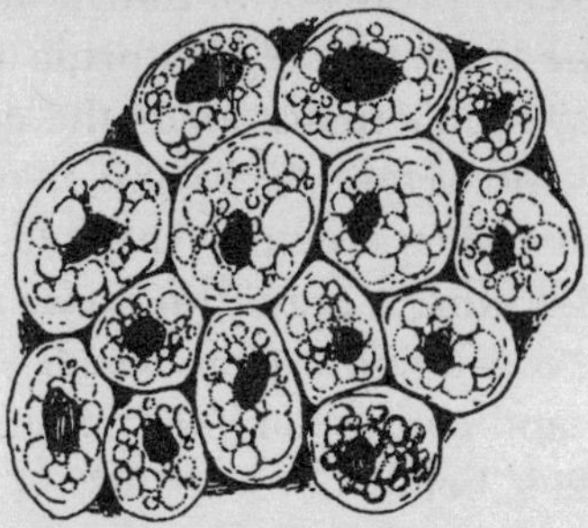

Figure 2. Fat cells — bubbles that hold extra calories.

maintaining a certain weight. If you feed them too much, they'll get fat. But as soon as they return to regular amounts of food, they return to their normal size. Likewise, if you starve them, they'll lose weight temporarily but quickly regain the lost pounds once they return to their old diets. Scientists refer to the weight level animals return to as their "set point."

If you think about it, the same is true with many people. Given a high-calorie diet, we gain weight until we return to less fattening food. And once we stop a low-calorie diet, we quickly regain the weight we've lost. In other words, people have set points, too.

The reason we have set points, say two Rockefeller University researchers, is that fat cells help dictate them. Drs. Rudolph Leibel and Jules Hirsch believe that our body's attempt to keep constant the size of its fat cells is what controls our desire to eat.

The scientists base that belief on what happens once they hospitalize very large people to reduce their weight to normal. "We discover an astonishing thing. They are not normal," Hirsch told *Science* magazine. After the weight loss, the once-obese patients somehow need 25 percent fewer calories than usual. So if they ate like they usually do, they'd gain weight. Conversely, once normal volunteers gain weight, they start to burn more calories. It's as if the body compensates for the amount of food it receives, adjusting its metabolism in an effort to return fat cells to their rightful size and body weight back to its magical set point.

At the root of this balancing act may be biochemical messages broadcast by the fat cells themselves. Fat people, whose fat cells are twice as large as usual, may be under the influence of messages that have gone awry, signaling them to overeat.

Theory 5: Not Enough Nerve Messengers

Nervous systems have been called the most intricately organized structures on earth. The nerve cells inside the human body connect each fingertip, each hair, each part of every organ with the brain and spinal cord, stretching throughout our anatomy like so many linking hands. Each of us has billions of nerve cells, and to get their job done, they must communicate with each other. For that task, nature in its ingenuity has provided chemical messengers known as *neurotransmitters*. One such neurotransmitter is *serotonin*. Produced inside the brain, serotonin is believed to play a role in regulating depression, sleep, and even symptoms of premenstrual tension. It's also thought to be tied to a person's weight.

At MIT, Professor Richard Wurtman was studying college students' diets when he noticed a puzzling trend. Given the choice between high-protein snacks and high-carbohydrate snacks, fat students consistently chose carbohydrates. Wurtman knew that carbohydrates act as a sort of fuel to help the brain manufacture serotonin and that, in fact, it's quite normal for people to crave carbohydrates from time to time, perhaps as a way of their bodies signaling a need for serotonin. But he also knew that most people have a self-regulating shutoff system, so that rising levels of serotonin eliminate our appetite for carbohydrates. "Presumably it keeps the bear from eating only honey and keeps human beings from eating sweets and starches to the exclusion of enough protein," says Wurtman. For some reason, the obese students were like a bear on a honey binge—they simply couldn't get enough carbos.

The answer, Wurtman reasoned, was that the students were failing to manufacture enough serotonin. As a result, their shutoff systems were never activated. Once the students were given a drug called fenfluramine, which increases serotonin levels, they cut down on carbohydrate-rich snacking and reduced the amount of carbohydrates they ate with meals. Serotonin-boosters may one day serve as a tool for weight loss. Until then, overweight people might take some comfort in knowing that their cravings for starches and sweets may well be biological, not just psychological.

Theory 6: Abnormal "Satiety Chemicals"

Want to trick someone into thinking they've had enough to eat? Just sprinkle a little GLP-1 into their corn flakes.

That's the theory, at least, that's been driving English researchers who are excited about the discovery of what could turn out to be an antiobesity hormone. GLP-1 is made in the lower reaches of the brain in response to as-yet-unknown signals from the body. Then it's transported to the hypothalamus gland, the body's main appetite control center. The stuff seems to really do a number on appetite. When it was injected into the brains of rats, their appetite dropped by 95 percent and they sat back and relaxed, just like they do after a big meal.

Researchers suspect GLP-1 could do for obesity what the discovery of aspirin did for headaches. But drug companies aren't waiting around to find out. No fewer than forty-five companies around the world are vying to be the first to finish research on one anti-obesity medication or the other. "It's potentially the world's biggest market for a drug," one researcher told the *Washington Post.*

Many of these experts are riding a wave of recent discoveries about so-called "satiety chemicals"—substances that tell us we've had enough to eat.

The first such substance to make headlines was the 1994 discovery of a hormone called leptin. Leptin is a natural appetite suppressant that's released by the body's fat cells. After a meal, newly plumped-up fat cells release leptin, which appears to signal our brain to push away from the table. This will give you an idea of how powerful leptin is: If you give leptin to a mouse that's genetically programmed to be hugely overweight, the hormone will completely negate its genes and the mouse's body weight will be no different from that of a mouse with normal genes.

Since that first breakthrough, scientists have speculated that abnormalities in the working of these and other chemicals might be responsible for obesity. For instance, fat people might have too little GLP-1, or might be unresponsive to it.

Theory 7: Stronger Reactions to Food

You've just arrived in a new town and you're hungry. So you stop the first black person you see and ask where to get a good bite to eat. It they're thin, they might name one or two nearby restaurants and keep going. But if they're fat, you may be in for a fervent description of area eateries, complete with a commentary on specific dishes. ("Now, the beef tip dinner at Smith's is great and the rolls are nice and hot. And don't forget the pecan pie. I like mine with a scoop of vanilla ice cream and a cup of coffee.")

If you've ever felt that eating is a fat person's favorite thing to do, you may be correct. Obesity experts tell us that obese people feel unusually connected to food. A meal that a thin person finds merely enjoyable may to a fat person seem thoroughly captivating in ways that only another fat person can truly understand.

"There's a theory that people who are obese are more cued in to food. They have a more intense reaction to external cues," Dr. Regina Casper, head of the eating disorders program at Chicago's Michael Reese Hospital, explained to a *Chicago Tribune* reporter. "You and I may pass a bakery and enjoy the aroma but keep going. However, obese people who pass a bakery may be unable to get food off their minds. They'll often go back and buy doughnuts."

Dr. Susan Schiffman, director of Duke University's obesity clinic, says that eighteen years of research have convinced her that people with various eating disorders have strong and very different food preferences and that fat people have a much greater need for texture and flavor. Put a bowl of whipped cream before a person with anorexia nervosa and they'll be repulsed, because anorexics hate fatty food. Put the same bowl before a fat person, and they'll be delighted. "The amounts of taste, smell, and texture needed to satisfy the overweight are much greater," Schiffman told the *Chicago Tribune.* "They crave crunch, elasticity, creaminess."

Schiffman has experimented for years with foods that recreate the sensory cues that fat people crave without dosing the diner with fat and calories. One creation: a bowl of strawberries topped with low-calorie chocolate powder, a sugar substitute, and a high-fiber cereal. Presto! Crunchiness, sweetness, and the sensuousness of chocolate—all for just 30 calories. She has developed hundreds of flavor packets that contain the essence of the fattening foods (cheese, butter, bacon, etc.) in a low-calorie powder that can be sprinkled over baked potatoes, broccoli, popcorn, you name it. These Flavor Enhancers, as they're called, are among the many weight-loss products available to clients at Nutri/System, Inc., weight-reduction centers, which number 1,500 nationwide.

ENVIRONMENTAL REASONS FOR FATNESS

With some people, body weight isn't as much physiological destiny as it is a product of our surroundings. Our cultural standards, our eating habits, our lifestyles and past experiences, our jobs and home lives—these are just some of the factors that combine to influence our body weight. Even geography plays a part. In 1997, a coalition of health and nutrition groups announced that our chances of being obese depend in part on where we live. In Denver, where people are "outdoorsy" and like to camp and hike, only 22 percent of the population is obese. In New Orleans, on the other hand, a 38 percent obese city renowned for its rich gumbos and sugary beignets, folks don't exercise much—partly because it rains a lot. Let's examine these nonbiological links between environment and body weight.

Cultural Standards

On the whole, Americans consider obesity about as popular as baldness, body odor, and bad breath combined. American culture teaches avoidance of fat and near-worship of lean, thin bodies.

Many Africans, on the other hand, are more tolerant of fatness, particularly in women. Across the continent and much of the rest of the nonindustrialized world, being fat means prosperity, health, and fertility (sometimes because thinness is a sign of starvation). In parts of Kenya, where a bridegroom's parents pay for the privilege of marriage, plump brides command higher prices than do skinny ones. Among the Amhara tribe of the Horn of Africa, calling a thin woman "dog hips" is a common insult.

When Africans become Westernized, many no longer adhere to this traditional view. Genevieve Ekaete of Howard University confided in *Essence* magazine that when she left Nigeria, her mother, "who among her native people in the eastern part of Nigeria would not be considered fat enough," asked the daughter to send her a supply of girdles. "She was, at the time, living in Lagos [Nigeria's Westernized capital city] and felt unattractive because she wasn't thin." Similarly, African-Americans may find themselves caught between two cultural norms—the African standard that appreciates a little extra padding, and the American standard that celebrates boyish thinness—even in women.

Many resolve this dilemma by going with their roots. "Black churchgoers think nothing of saving an extra large space on the pew for Sister So-and-So," says Dr. Shiriki Kumanyika, a Pennsylvania State University researcher who specializes in obesity and African-Americans. Ardena Shankar, a professional personnel consultant and chair of the Santa Cruz County (CA) Task Force on Self-Esteem, says she has always felt that her weight is less of an issue among blacks than among whites. "Our community is much more accepting of fat people. Black people seem to be able to judge a fat person for who they are rather than superficialities like what size they are."

Black folks have also been dosed by years of exposure to the "mammy" image. From actresses like Oscar-winning Hattie McDaniel and 1950s television star Louise Beavers to the modern-day Nell Carter, American culture continues to cast fat black women in the role of irascible but lovable maids. The image is so popular and ingrained that a mammy appears in one of the oldest trademarks in America—Aunt Jemima's pancake mix, which was first marketed in 1889. Can any child not be comforted by these smiling images of hefty black women? They are images we have been conditioned to embrace. Dr. Deborah Dawson of the National Center for Health Statistics, who has studied ethnic differences in women's perceptions of their weight, says that black women are less likely than white women to perceive themselves as overweight. But when you ask black women to compare their weight against other black women, the response is about the same as when white women are asked to compare themselves with their white peers. In other words, the heavier a woman's peers are, the more latitude she may feel to gain weight herself without risking social isolation. That could be one additional explanation for why black folks are heavier than whites.

African-Americans may also be more accepting of the health problems that stem from being fat. When our elders develop such severe arthritis that they cannot comfortably climb the church stairs, we take it in stride and install an elevator. When our relatives get progressively sicker with diabetes and end up on dialysis, we tell ourselves it's the Lord's will. One black woman proudly told researcher Dr. Shiriki Kumanyika, "My family has diabetes so bad that people say you're not a member of the family unless your toes fall off when you get older." Recalls Kumanyika, "I was shocked at how casually this highly educated woman and her family had accepted this terrible disease." You can see that loving our community and cherishing our families—two traditional strong points for black people—doesn't always lead to good health.

Still, body weight for black Americans can bring up difficult choices. We who are African by ancestry but American by birth are socialized early on to accept prevailing standards of beauty. For well over a century, we've straightened our hair and bleached our skin in a quiet, desperate attempt to circumvent color-based rejection by whites. Why should we consider our weight any differently? Indeed, sociologist Dr. Becky Wangsgaard Thompson, who has worked with women of color who have eating disorders, suspects that the acceptance of prevailing standards of weight might ironically explain why black women are so heavy. "It's a well-known fact that dieting makes a person gain weight," Thompson explains. "Black women may diet repeatedly but not very openly, because they feel that dieting is something white women do." If Thompson is correct, one reason we weigh what we do may have more to do with our bowing to American standards than embracing African ones.

Sedentary Lifestyle

Appliance makers are fond of advertising how efficiently their devices operate. Why, you can run this fan or that vacuum cleaner for only pennies a year, they say. What they don't mention is that there's a hidden cost to all of these many food processors and hedge clippers. What may seem like savings in your wallet may turn out to be sabotage for your waistline.

Psychologist Dr. Thomas Wadden of the University of Pennsylvania School of Medicine says the problem with all of these labor-saving devices is that, to put it bluntly, they save labor. And when we rely on machines instead of our muscles, we lose out on the chance to burn a few calories.

How much harm can a little convenience cause, you might wonder? If you were to ditch your extension phone, you would walk an additional 70 miles per year, on average. That's the equivalent of 2 pounds of fat. Would you consider trading in your desktop computer for a manual typewriter? You'd lose an additional 4 pounds of body fat. And let's not talk about the more substantial work savers in our lives, like cars and buses. Can you imagine how many pounds we gain as a nation each year for the privilege of retiring our walking shoes, letting our bicycles rust, and reclining in splendor while a 2-ton box of metal and glass glides us anywhere we want to go?

There's no question that America's sedentary lifestyle contributes to our weight problem. As a nation, we consume anywhere from 3 to 10 percent fewer calories than we did in 1900. Yet there's twice as much obesity now than there was then.

Our African-American grandparents' grandparents didn't choose their lifestyle as much as it was thrust upon them. But for all of the barbarity that slavery was, and for all of the hardship endured by black farmers and laborers and factory workers after the Civil War, black people never had to think about getting exercise. We *lived* exercise. Today, the calories that once went into walking to the field to pick cotton now go into driving to the mall to pick designer cotton fashions. Surveys show that black Americans get less exercise than whites do, whether it's climbing stairs, participating in sports, working in a garden, or simply walking.

Eating Habits

Granted African-Americans get less than our share of exercise. Do we come up short on our eating habits, too? Not necessarily. Make no mistake—we could certainly stand to improve the typical African-American diet, which is laced with sodium, fat, and sugar, and low in whole grains and fresh fruits and vegetables. But on the whole, although African-Americans are heavier than whites, black people actually consume about the same number of calories as white people do. (One exception is black teenage girls, who eat more than their white counterparts.

This may be important because obesity in black females often begins during adolescence.)

Our eating habits can tell disturbing truths about us, however, because obesity, and the overeating that can lead to it, can be a sign of distress. "White feminists usually explain fatness by pointing to gender inequality, and the frustration and rage that women feel in a male-dominated world," explains Dr. Becky Wangsgaard Thompson. That may be true; American standards of attractiveness are stricter for women, and it's still much harder for women to command the same respect as men. "But my research suggests that discrimination based on race, class, poverty, and sexual orientation can play a major role, particularly in the African-American community. To the extent that these factors affect black males, boys and men can develop problematic relationships with food just as women can."

In some cases, we eat as a way of coping with a painful past. "Children who live in a world in which adverse circumstances exist based on the color of their skin and ethnicity are constantly confronted with circumstances that they had no hand in creating," writes Claudia Black, a founder of the Adult Children of Alcoholics movement. Among the many circumstances that confront African-American children are parental and familial abuse—drug abuse (including alcoholism), sexual abuse (including incest), physical abuse, and emotional abuse. All of it is more common in families under stress. In that category black families are overrepresented, since we are disproportionately unemployed, undervalued, undereducated, uninsured, and underrespected. One manifestation of growing up in an abusive situation? Eating disorders.

According to psychiatrists, studies show that most overweight people are no more psychologically disturbed than are people who weigh less. Obesity isn't *necessarily* the result of an eating disorder, any more than thinness is. But for children as well as adults who have endured abuse as a child, and for adults whose present lives are tumultuous, eating can become a compulsion that helps block out unpleasant reminders and anesthetize them against the pain. Byllye Avery, founding president of the National Black Women's Health Project, recalls one obese black woman who explained her weight with crystal clarity. "My old man is an alcoholic. My kid's got babies. One thing I know I can do when I come home is cook me a pot of food and sit in front of the TV and eat it."

For youngsters whose lives are careening out of control, eating can also symbolize a way to bring order to chaos. Faced with a violent, unpredictable home life, replete with alcoholism or physical or sexual assault, plus a difficult school life that may involve racist abuse from teachers or classmates, some black children may decide that the only area of their lives that they can control is what they put into their mouths. The results can range from overeating to food obsessions, or even to their opposite with anorexia nervosa—self-induced starvation.

For people who are depressed or whose lives lack love, food can become a substitute for the emotional sustenance they crave. "All too often people are not eating for nutrition. Rather, they're eating for comfort," suggests Washington State University nutrition expert Gladys Pullman in *Essence* magazine. Claudia Black agrees. "People who feel poorly about themselves often use food for solace. Those with low self-esteem and a tendency to isolate themselves are much more likely to regard food as a friend."

Fat people may eat out of fear. If you've never been cared for, you may fear abandonment. If you're an incest survivor, you may fear looking sexy. If you've been physically abused, you may fear being attacked again, so you gain weight to give you the strength to fight back. "I wasn't always fat," recalls Ardena Shankar. "I was a thin child until I started getting molested. My weight just took off after that."

The more we use food to try to satisfy nonphysical needs, the harder it becomes to recognize our body's genuine hunger cues. Eventually, we no longer distinguish between physical needs and emotional ones. We're on the path to an eating disorder.

How to Get Help for Problem Eating

If you want to lose weight, literally thousands of commercial diet centers across the country will be all too willing to lighten your wallet. But if you want to get to the bottom of an unhealthy relationship with food—and there's a difference—these establishments may not be of much use. One weight-loss program makes clients wear dunce caps if they have gained weight since the previous meeting. That's hardly constructive. The philosophy of weight-loss programs differs from one company to the next, but any given organization may not have the expertise—or the interest, frankly—in helping you get at the deeper reasons for why your eating behavior is so problematic. After all, they make money when people diet, not when people resolve an eating disorder and stop coming.

Here are some suggestions from sociologist Dr. Becky Wangsgaard Thompson. Start by educating yourself about what eating disorders are and how to recognize them. For an excellent guide to childhood sexual abuse, which is one cause of eating disorders, see *The Courage to Heal: A Guide for Women Survivors of Child Sexual Abuse* by Ellen Bass and Laura Davis (HarperCollins, 1994) and *The Courage to Heal Workbook* by

Laura Davis (HarperCollins, 1990). For fictional reading, the central character in novelist Toni Morrison's *The Bluest Eye* dissociates from her body so completely—a common experience in child abuse—that all that's left are her eyes.

Women with eating disorders often say that joining any self-help group is immensely helpful. Whether fighting for tenant rights, advocating for battered women, or celebrating sexual preference, organizations that help women come together and recognize their collective strengths often help members realize their own individual strengths as well, because eating disorders are often symptoms of a larger sense of feeling disempowered.

You may find that you need counseling to help sort things out. Free or low-cost counseling is available at community mental health clinics and some hospital- or clinic-based weight-loss programs in many areas of the country. Two of the more popular organizations that include counseling in their work are Overeaters Anonymous and Weight Watchers International. Overeaters Anonymous helps members control compulsive eating by engendering self-esteem and providing a supportive network of fellow overeaters. It is based on a twelve-step approach to facing addictions. The organization claims over 120,000 members worldwide. Membership is free. The only requirement is a desire to stop eating compulsively. To locate a group near you, check the white pages of your phone book or contact:

Overeaters Anonymous
6075 Zenith Court N.E.
Rio Rancho, NM 87124-6424
(505) 891-2664
Web site: www.overeatersAnonymous.org
E-mail: overeatr@technet.nm.org

Weight Watchers International combines nutritious food plans with low- to moderate-intensity exercise, group support, and a behavioral management plan. The program uses either preplanned menus or extensive food lists, depending on whether members prefer a structured eating prescription or more latitude to choose their own meals. A maintenance program is available once members reach their individual goals by gradually losing 1 to 2 pounds per week. In recent years Weight Watchers has shifted its emphasis from counting calories or food exchanges to counting points. Allowable points are decided on an individual basis. To reach Weight Watchers, check the white pages of your phone book or contact:

Weight Watchers International, Inc.
c/o Lelio Parduzzi
175 Crossways Park West
N. Woodbury, NY 11797-2055
(516) 390-1400
Web site: www.weightwatchers.com

CHAPTER 4

The Truth About Dieting

Losing weight, and keeping it off, can be one of the most agonizing personal struggles a person will ever endure. Ask Oprah Winfrey.

Oprah may look radiant and slender-chic as she smiles from the covers of half of the women's magazines in your supermarket checkout line. But she'll be the first to tell you that behind the smile lie years of anguish over her weight.

In 1988, the celebrated talk-show hostess decided that she was fed up. Fed up with trying and discarding every new diet that came along. Fed up with feeling her self-esteem stymied by fat—"like having mud in my wings" is how she described it in her journal. Fed up with seven years of weight-loss regimens that left her seventy pounds *heavier* than when she began. She tried every conventional approach, and every conventional approach had failed her.

So she decided to play hardball. She had heard of a liquid protein diet called Optifast. The new diet was doctor-supervised, and people who had tried it had lost lots of weight. What did she have to lose?

Every day, Oprah Winfrey stirred five packets of powder into a glass of water and drank. And at the end of four months, she stepped before a national television audience to reveal something she had been dreaming of for the better part of a decade: a brand new body. Clad in a black turtleneck and the size-10 jeans she had always fantasized wearing, Oprah danced around the stage to the cheers of her audience. She had lost 67 pounds. She even wheeled out 67 pounds of animal fat to drive home the significance. "I can't lift it, but I used to carry it around every day," she said. It was an exciting moment for the many who knew of Oprah's painful history as an incest survivor and of her long struggle to come to terms with her weight.

But before long, the cheers turned to dismay. Week by week, slowly but surely, the pounds were returning. Everyone saw it. Everyone watched as the designer jeans gave way to roomier dresses. Finally, after a two-year struggle to maintain the weight loss she had so desperately craved, Oprah Winfrey told America that her battle with her weight was over. Having once basked in what she termed "the single greatest accomplishment of my life," Oprah Winfrey simply gave up trying to be someone she wasn't. "My greatest failure was in believing that the weight issue was just about weight," she told *People* magazine. "It's not." For Oprah, the real challenge was handling stresses in a way that's healthy rather than self-destructive.

Oprah has since lost a significant amount of weight, thanks to a plan that combines smart eating with vigorous exercise. She admits that she hasn't yet fallen into a comfortable rhythm on the exercise, though it's a crucial element of her success with achieving—and maintaining—her present weight.

Folks from coast to coast are cheering for Oprah, because millions of us can relate to her story. In our own desperation to lose weight, for example, we spend billions a year on commercial diet plans, over-the-counter diet drugs, and vitamins, all in the hope that *this* diet (whichever one we happen to be on) will be the one that triumphs. But what many of us understand from experience, doctors and nutritionists know from careful research: *Most diets fail.* They fail because it's much easier to take pounds off than it is to keep them off.

Losing the weight means making a temporary change in behavior—forgoing snacks for a while, giving up desserts for a couple of months, crunching carrot sticks through a movie instead of reaching for hot buttered popcorn. Keeping it off means making permanent changes in lifestyle—and that's a lot harder. Thus, the huge majority of all diets go up in smoke.

Roughly 90 percent of all dieters who lose 25 pounds regain them within two years, according to the National Center for Health Statistics. And only 2 percent of all dieters who manage to achieve their desired weight maintain it for seven years. Many even wind up weighing more than they did before they started their diets! As one researcher admits, "Now we're even asking the question, 'Does dieting *cause* obesity?'"

It's pretty sobering stuff, this talk about the apparent futility of even trying to lose weight. But don't despair. There *are* answers. There are reasons that some people manage to lose weight and keep it off. To place these solutions in context, though, let's first take a broader look at some of the biological mechanisms that explain why successful dieting is easier said than done.

THE BIOLOGY OF DIETING

Let yourself travel back hundreds of years and imagine for a moment your ancestors on the continent. For the most part, their food supply is adequate. But when they lose part of their crops to bad weather, or there's a lull in the hunting, things can get lean. The people who survive are those who can save food when it's plentiful, and subsist on it when food is scarce. For our ancestors, fat became the key to survival. Once food satisfies the body's immediate needs, any extra calories get converted to fat, which in turn becomes a source of energy when the going gets rough. Over time, this ability to store fat is passed genetically from generation to generation, and makes a key contribution to the survival of the race.

Now picture African-Americans today. Despite being surrounded by food that's immensely more plentiful—and more fattening—many of us are just five or six generations removed from Africa. In evolutionary terms, that's a mere blink of the eye, not nearly enough time for our genes to change very much. And those genes tell our bodies to hang on to every extra calorie, because we might need it later. That's one theory behind why it's much easier for us to gain weight than to lose it; our bodies are programmed to accumulate.

African-Americans aren't the only folks influenced by calorie-collecting genes. Everyone has a built-in drive to conserve calories. Around the globe, populations who suddenly find themselves swamped with food start to get fat. (Remember the Chinese weight-loss clinic described in Chapter 2?)

So even before you embark on a weight-loss program, you've got imbedded inside you strong biological urges running in the opposite direction. Now, once you actually start to diet, additional factors come into play. For instance, you've probably noticed that when you diet, you lose a fair amount of weight in the first week or two. You flush with pride. Suddenly, your life as a thin person doesn't seem all that impossible after all. But that hopeful sense of accomplishment soon starts to slip through your fingers. As the days go on, you lose less and less with each passing week. Enthusiasm has melted to disappointment.

Don't feel bad. It happens to everyone. The human body reacts to food deprivation by conserving calories. It's another survival mechanism: Your body wants to protect you from starvation, even though your mind may know full well that you have a refrigerator full of food. Your body begins to conserve calories, faithfully protecting you from a threat that will never materialize. Suddenly your smooth-running diet machine is out of gas.

Here's an example. Let's suppose that you eat 2,000 calories a day, and that your metabolism burns 2,000 calories a day. Your weight is stable; your body chemistry is such that when you eat the same number of calories that you burn, you neither gain weight nor lose it. But you decide that you're subjecting your favorite pants to cruel and unusual punishment, so you go to a diet that allows only 1,000 calories per day. Since you're now burning up more than you're eating, you start to lose weight. But not for long, because your body reacts by conserving calories. Soon it burns only 1,800 calories per day, then 1,500. Before long, you're burning 1,000 calories— exactly what you take in. And your weight loss stops.

At your new lighter weight, you may have once

again made friends with your wardrobe. But you're faced with two new dilemmas. First of all, you can't eat as much as you originally could without gaining weight. At first, your body was used to burning 2,000 calories—twice as much as your new metabolism allows. Now you have less room for error, because if you eat more than 1,000 calories a day, you'll start to put on the pounds again.

The second hitch is that if you happen to abandon your diet, your metabolic rate will eventually return to its original level of 2,000 calories a day. No harm there. But if you step off and on the diet bandwagon enough times, your metabolism could get stuck at the lower level. In other words, if you try a 1,000-calorie diet enough times, you could end up burning 1,000 calories a day no matter what you eat. This is what happens with so-called yo-yo dieting, and it helps explain why chronic dieters often complain that repeated dieting actually makes them gain weight.

What Goes Down Must Come Up: The Hazards of Yo-Yo Dieting

On any given day, fully one-quarter of all overweight American men—and half of all overweight women—are on a diet. And many of those people diet for years at a time. You know the pattern. You gain weight each winter, and go on a crash diet to fit into your swimsuit each spring. Or you lose weight with one diet but eventually give it up (and gain back the weight you lost, plus more), only to seize on the next new diet that happens to come along. Many dieters don't realize that such fluctuating weight changes can cause a number of counterproductive side effects:

- *Heart disease.* Yo-yo dieting increases the risk of heart disease, perhaps because it redistributes fat, often from the hips to the belly. Abdominal fat cells seem to release fat into the bloodstream more readily than do fat cells in the thighs or hips—one reason that belly fat is believed riskier to the heart.

- *Weight gain.* Repeated dieting tends to lower the body's metabolic rate, which means you burn fewer calories. That leads to eventual weight gain. If a person's weight is already cause for health concern, imagine the dangers of heightening the risks ever further.
- *Less lean, more fat.* On-again, off-again dieting changes the body's tissue composition, so that people end up with more fat and less lean than before. Yo-yo dieters also tend to eat fattier foods. That not only leads to more weight gain, but also increases the risk of heart disease and cancers of the breast and colon.

When you add it all up, you can see why one obesity researcher says, "Being overweight is serious, but we seem to be finding a greater risk if you're fluctuating. This yo-yo dieting is a major concern."

There's one more way that human biology thwarts diets. When fat people lose weight, their bodies produce an enzyme that makes it easy to gain weight again.

Weight loss drains the fat from a person's fat cells, which shrink. But in hefty people, weight loss also triggers the overproduction of an enzyme called *lipoprotein lipase.* The enzyme puffs up the depleted fat cells, making it easier for them to start filling with fat again.

If you're not on a diet, lipoprotein lipase doesn't make you gain weight, although scientists think the enzyme does help fat people maintain their weight. It's when people lose weight that the action really begins. Enzyme factories throughout the body kick into high gear, churning out doses of lipoprotein lipase that head straight for the now-depleted fat cells. The heavier you are, the more enzyme your body produces after weight loss—and the more your shrunken fat cells get primed to refill with fat. Lipoprotein lipase helps explain why everyone seems to have a set point, a certain weight that the body prefers. "If you believe in set points, it's not hard to imagine that the body would defend itself against weight loss," explained one obesity researcher when new findings about the enzyme were announced back in 1990. "As weight goes down, you reach a level that sets the body in motion to restore the lost weight. Maybe these findings about lipoprotein levels explain why that occurs."

No wonder dieters have trouble maintaining their new weight! Their enzymes are scrambling to regain every lost ounce. "It's so consistent with what our patients tell us," obesity specialist Dr. Adam Drewnowski told the *New York Times*. "Many of our patients report that in order to maintain a reduced weight, they need to eat almost nothing and, in some cases, to exercise at very high levels." (We'll examine the importance of exercise in Chapter 5.)

When you put it all together, you can end up with a powerful argument that diets are destined to flop. With our survival-minded bodies conserving against weight loss to begin with, then fighting to regain any weight that we manage to lose, dieting may seem about as promising as trying to squeeze a size 14D foot into a size 6A shoe.

It's not very surprising that fat people give up on diets altogether. For one thing, the dieting process itself is often physically excruciating. Substantial weight loss often leaves a person chronically tired and cold (remember how dieting slows down your metabolism?). Formerly fat women who lose a great deal of weight often stop menstruating and can't get pregnant.

The psychological toll is substantial, too. Dieters face a constant temptation to eat—by glorious full-color television commercials, mouth-watering lunches carried to work by nondieters, aromas wafting from bakeries and pizza parlors and fried-chicken joints. Dieters find they spend a substantial amount of energy simply keeping themselves motivated to maintain a weight that naturally thin people take for granted.

Harvard Medical School obesity expert Dr. George Blackburn estimates that at least half of all fat people who try to achieve their desirable weight (according to insurance-company charts) suffer medical, physical, and psychological complications. That's why even some fat people who can lose weight and keep it off say that dieting just isn't for them.

Does Dieting Make You Pig Out?

Who eats more — a person who's watching their weight, or someone who isn't? The surprising answer came to light at Northwestern University, where scientists asked groups of dieters and nondieters first to taste some milkshakes, then to eat as much as they wanted from a large dish of ice cream.

The more milkshakes that the nondieters drank, the less ice cream they wanted afterwards. After all, ice cream and shakes are great-tasting treats, but a person can only take so much.

But the dieters' experience was completely different. After two milkshakes, they ate more ice cream than if they drank none or one. Their appetite for ice cream wasn't diminished by the milkshakes. It was increased!

What happened? The dieters felt that they could safely indulge in one milkshake and still stick to their diets. But anything more than that represented crossing a line. Once these normally controlled eaters torpedoed their diets by slurping up two milkshakes, they gave up trying to restrain themselves and simply went for broke.

Moral: When it comes to eating, conscious restraint is a fragile thing.

And yet many of us can't afford *not* to lose weight. Our size simply makes our lives too difficult, adding a thick layer of distress to a daily existence already made stressful enough by the multiple challenges of being black in America. Not to mention the health concerns. Millions of us risk burdening our hearts, heightening our chance of cancer, raising our blood pressure, and ultimately shortening our lives.

Those of us who've abandoned every diet that we've tried may have more than once felt the temptation to resort to stronger medicine.

REACHING FOR A PILL

Once we unload our diet books at the first available garage sale, the next line of defense for many of us is a distinctly American solution: We reach for a pill. We take pills to keep our pressure under control, right? Why not take them to keep our weight under control?

Well, there are a few things you should know about weight-loss pills. Many over-the-counter weight-loss medicines contain a compound called phenylpropanolamine (PPA for short). PPA is a stimulant that can push up your blood pressure, so it's not the best stuff to have in your system if you, like many black folks, have high blood pressure to begin with. The drug has also been linked in rare cases to strokelike symptoms, according to the Center for the Science in the Public Interest (CSPI), a Washington, D.C., consumer group. And while some people who take PPA may experience significant weight loss, most do not, says CSPI.

What about prescription medicines? You may remember the alarm in 1997 over "fen/phen," a combination of the weight-loss drugs fenfluramine and phentermine. In the 1990s doctors started prescribing these medicines together, rather than the separate uses FDA had envisioned when it approved them. The extra potency made fen/phen a popular favorite at commercial diet centers until people realized that the combination could damage a person's heart valves. The two drugs were pulled from the market shortly thereafter.

One of the more recent prescription weight-loss drugs to hit the market is called Meridia. It works by elevating levels of a brain chemical that causes you to feel full. Unlike PPA, Meridia really seems to work. Ellen Wallen of Janesville, Wisconsin, a lifelong dieter and exerciser, used to have such a craving for greasy fast food that she'd hit the drive-through for lunch, head home for a nap, hit it again on the return trip to work, then visit a third time at the end of the day. With Meridia, she can drive past Taco Bell without stopping. "It removes that sense of desperation to eat," she told the *Washington Post.* Most other prescription drugs are either amphetamines or amphetamine-like, and like PPA, they spike your blood pressure. Translation: Tread lightly.

The real buzz in the pharmaceutical industry these days is over a slew of antiobesity compounds that are in the research pipeline. Two of the hopefuls are leptin and GLP-1, which you may remember from the previous chapter. Pfizer, the drug company that brought us the anti-impotence drug Viagra, is working on a medicine that will block the action of a natural substance called neuropeptide Y that seems to make experimental animals hungry. Hoffmann-LaRoche, the Swiss pharmaceutical firm, is making a drug called Xenical, which is supposed to help you lose weight by stopping fat from being absorbed by the intestines. People who take it absorb about one-third less fat than without the medicine. Xenical is already selling—and selling well—in Europe and parts of Asia. Other drug firms are working on ways to rev up the body's metabolism so we burn more calories.

None of these experimental medicines have been approved by the U.S. Food and Drug Administration, so it's too early to tell exactly how safe—or effective—they are. Already, though, researchers do know that Xenical, the fat blocker, can cause intestinal distress in some people and, more seriously, may raise the risk of breast cancer in women. If and when the new wonder drugs make it to the corner drugstore, the best advice is to work with your doctor to carefully weigh the risks and benefits. For example, Meridia, the drug that helps you feel full, shouldn't be taken if you have heart disease because, like PPA, it can raise your blood pressure and make your heart race. On the other hand, unlike PPA, when you combine the medicine with exercise and a good diet, many people can lose 10 percent of their body weight. If you haven't been able to lose weight despite eating carefully and exercising persistently, and you're in good cardiovascular health, Meridia might be a sensible option. Ask your doctor.

GOING SURGICAL

In the last two decades, growing numbers of Americans have opted for the most extreme weight-loss option—going under the knife. You may have heard of some of these approaches, wondered what they're about, and especially wondered if they work. Let's review the options. If you're willing to take the risks, and you can afford it, you have four major alternatives. You can *build a detour, trick your tummy, suck it out, or starve it off.*

Building a Detour

As troublesome as it can be when it grows a little too big for our shirts, the human abdomen—and what goes on inside it—are unsung heroes. First, there's the stomach, a tidy little collection center where the food we swallow gets churned up with enzymes and other digestive juices. These liquids help break down each mouthful of our last meal into simpler nutrients that the body can absorb. Most of the absorption happens in the next phase of the process when the partially digested food passes into the small intestine. This is essentially a tube, the inside wall of which is covered by microscopic fingerlike projections called *villi.* Through the villi pass the many nutrients that keep us alive.

Many people don't realize how efficiently this digestive arrangement works. To begin with, the small intestine is only 1½ inches in diameter, but it's 20 to 25 feet long. What's more, the villi give the intestine an enormous surface area. In fact, if the intestine were to lie completely flat, it would cover more than 300 square yards—about the size of a tennis court. In the early 1970s, doctors started wondering if they could help fat people lose weight by cutting that tennis court down to size. They figured that reducing the surface area of the digestive tract would allow less food to be absorbed, thus reducing the number of calories a person took into his or her body.

The first procedure to emerge from these deliberations was the *intestinal bypass,* in which surgeons attached the first few feet of the small intestine to the last few feet, thereby bypassing much of the intestine's length. Before long, there were problems. After an intestinal bypass in 1974, Mary-Jane Grace-Brown dropped from 450 to 140 pounds in nine months. But she had to be hospitalized for the complications that set in—severe malnutrition, kidney disease, hair loss, an enlarged heart. "By the time I was down to 140, my bones were so brittle, they were afraid for me to even step off a curb," she told an *Atlanta Constitution* reporter. "I was so sick that I finally checked into a hospital in 1979 and had the operation reversed." Few intestinal bypasses are performed nowadays, because of the tendency for such complications. In fact, for a while, intestinal bypass operations gave obesity surgery a bad reputation.

But the next generation of bypasses has been more successful. During a *gastric stomach bypass,* doctors attach a section of the small intestine directly to the stomach. That allows some food to take a detour past the stomach and part of the intestine, which reduces the amount of food that can be absorbed. In 1991, a fourteen-member National Institutes of Health panel recommended the stomach bypass as one of two surgical procedures that are safe and effective ways to lose weight. (But read on for some important cautions.)

Tricking Your Tummy

The second NIH-recommended procedure involves a bit of willful deception. One of the reasons that people gain weight is that for one reason or another, they have a difficult time feeling full. We get this sense of fullness from a chain reaction that starts in our abdomen, where food somehow triggers the release of hormones that tell our brains that we no longer need to eat. Since the hormones are normally dispatched when our stomachs are full of food, enterprising surgeons wondered what would happen if they simply made the stomach smaller, enabling it to fill with less food. Thus was born stomach stapling, a surgical procedure that artificially shrinks the stomach to a fraction of its former size.

Stomach stapling closes off most of the stomach, creating a small pouch instead. A surgeon connects the small intestine to the pouch, and what results is essentially a "ministomach" that fills with food much faster than the original. As a result, patients feel full sooner and eat much less. Because the procedure cuts down on the amount of digestion that can take place, it also limits nutrient intake—a second way that stomach stapling curbs obesity.

Sucking It Out

In a culture that adores quick fixes, *liposuction* is the ultimate fantasy come true. Hate that weight? Suck it away. As operations go, it's a simple procedure. Once a patient is anesthetized, the surgeon inserts a hollow needle under the skin. The other end of the needle is connected to a vacuum pump, and when the switch is thrown, fat gets sucked right off the body.

Liposuction doesn't cure obesity, however. And it's only used for overweight patients in conjunction with other weight-loss procedures. In fact, most liposuction operations are performed for cosmetic reasons on people who are dissatisfied with their curves and bulges but who aren't fat.

Starving It Off

This is what Oprah tried during her early weight-loss disappointment. Today's liquid protein diet is quite a bit different from the over-the-counter liquid protein concoctions that led to at least seventeen deaths in the 1970s. Those preparations were based on vegetable proteins, while the modern version is made from the higher-quality proteins found in milk and egg white plus important minerals and vitamins. Alternatively, some of us are so determined to lose weight that we have our jaws wired shut. By the early 1990s, nearly a hundred such desperate dieters across the nation did so each day.

DO EXTREME PROBLEMS CALL FOR EXTREME SOLUTIONS?

Do these extreme weight-loss procedures make sense for African-Americans distressed about their weight? In most cases, the answer is no. Let's look at the three most important questions.

Are They Effective?

Scientists have doubts about the long-term effectiveness of drastic weight-management techniques. Recent evidence suggests that liquid protein diets don't seem to be any more effective for long-term weight loss than do carefully designed weight-loss programs that use regular food. For most people, stomach stapling and stomach bypass operations are effective for a year or

Do Liquid Protein Diets Work? An Expert's Opinion

In the old days, the world would beat a path to your door if you built a better mousetrap. Nowadays, all you have to do is peddle diet products. Americans spend billions on diet products every year. What we get for our money, says Oregon Congressman Ron Wyden, is "a tidal wave of false and misleading advertising in a field already awash in gross overpromotion." That's partly because the federal government doesn't regulate diet products very closely. It's also because no one has subjected diet products to careful testing. No one, that is, except Dr. Thomas Wadden, a psychologist and obesity expert with the University of Pennsylvania School of Medicine, who in 1992 published a study of the effectiveness of Optifast, a weight-loss product made famous by longtime dieter Oprah Winfrey.

Wadden studied several hundred men and women who, under a doctor's supervision, used Optifast liquid protein for six months before gradually returning to regular food. Patients also attended weekly meetings where they learned to keep food diaries, control unwanted eating, be assertive, and prevent relapses. The average patient weighed 233 pounds at the start of the study, and lost 50 pounds in the first six months.

That's the good news. The bad news is that nearly half of the dieters who started the program dropped out before the end of the twenty-six weeks. And when Wadden followed up on the patients after one year, he discovered that only 20 percent who had finished the program had managed to prevent their lost weight from returning. "This is certainly not a breakthrough in obesity treatment," Wadden told the *New York Times*, though he praised the makers of Optifast, Sandoz Nutrition Corporation, for allowing the study. "Now the rest of the diet industry has to come up with this kind of information."

Don't hold your breath, though. Diet companies are raking in money hand over fist. Until they're required by law to test their products, why should they risk spoiling a good thing?

two, according to NIH. After that a person may start to slowly regain lost weight. Until doctors conduct long-term follow-up studies on patients, the jury will remain out on the ultimate effectiveness of drastic weight-loss techniques. Given what we know about the body's tendency to return to its set point, it's a pretty safe bet that any weight loss, whether moderate or severe, is bound to be at least influenced by the same genetic drive for weight restoration that stymies more conventional dieters.

Are They Safe?

The risks vary. Many people who lose a great deal of weight suffer some side effects, including dizziness and sensitivity to cold, from the weight loss alone. The nature of other side effects and their severity can vary depending on the person, the procedure, and the skill and the experience of the physician who performs surgery or who monitors and advises a nonsurgical patient. Malnutrition after stomach stapling or stomach bypass surgery is common. Up to 10 percent of all patients risk problems ranging from abdominal disturbances (diarrhea, an uncomfortable feeling of fullness, or even an aversion to food) to staples coming undone, infection setting in, and bleeding into the abdomen. Stomach stapling also causes pain and nausea or vomiting if you eat too much. Protein-supplement fasting has not been linked with any deaths, although some fasters experience bad breath, dry skin, and other problems.

The risks of these procedures must be seen in perspective. Remember, carrying too much body weight is dangerous, too. For example, the risk of dying from stomach stapling or gastric bypass surgery is around 0.5 percent. In contrast, morbidly obese men die at a rate of 3 percent per year. If someone is so fat that losing weight is literally a matter of life and death and no other technique has worked, then surgery or fasting may be a lifesaver.

People Who *Shouldn't* Try to Lose Weight Without a Doctor's Supervision

- Severely fat people (your body weight could be a sign of an underlying illness that a doctor can discover)
- Pregnant or breastfeeding women
- Children
- Persons over the age of sixty-five
- Persons with medical conditions that make weight loss dangerous

Is It Worth the Cost?

Make no mistake—extreme treatments for obesity don't come cheap. Surgery costs thousands of dollars. Fasting can run $100 a week. Not many African-Americans can fork over that kind of money, and health insurance doesn't always cover the tab.

Despite federal approval, surgery for obesity is frowned on by many physicians except in the most extreme cases. The risks are too high, they say, and the payoff too uncertain. Fortunately, most obese African-Americans do not need the severest weight-reduction techniques. But many of us do need to lose weight. If dieting so often fails, what's the solution? *Is* there a solution?

Evidence from across the nation suggests that the answer is yes. In New Orleans, where low-income overweight black mothers exercise to the sounds of black music and learn about nutrition, participants lose weight and keep it off. In Atlanta, where a black urban community group has organized a club to use exercise and nutrition education to reduce the risk of heart disease, participants lose weight and lower their blood pressure. In Baltimore, where a church-based program teaches African-American women good food choices and low-impact aerobics, the women lose weight as they make permanent changes to their lifestyles.

When we make gradual but meaningful changes in our lifestyles, interesting things begin to happen. Granted our bodies, always vigilant for possible starvation, still resist weight change away from their set points. But when people combine nutritious eating with regular exercise, they often lose weight as a result. And a healthy lifestyle does wonders for more than our bodies. Our emotional health, our spiritual well-being, our intellectual power—all of these parts of us are enhanced as well. We'll learn the safest, most effective ways to achieve two of the most important lifestyle habits in the next two chapters.

CHAPTER 5

The "E" Word: An Important and Neglected Ally

Let's not beat around the bush: Most people hate to exercise. And most hefty people hate it even more. It's not that we doubt that exercise can do us good. It's just that exercise is…well, it's too much like work. Even more so for large bodies that may resist bending and that may hurt when joints are asked to support excess body weight. Exercise gets a bad rap from African-Americans for another reason, too: We assume it's something that only rich people have the money and time to do. "When we think of exercise, we think of clubs and membership fees," says Lisa White, national program developer for the National Black Women's Health Project, the Atlanta–based health-empowerment group. "And we assume that only the rich have enough leisure time to be able to spend their days exercising." So given the option of either watching a sport or participating in it, many of us waste no time deliberating. We just pull up an easy chair and tear open a bag of chips.

African-Americans have always had plenty of athletic role models; Arthur Ashe's *Hard Road to Glory,* a three-volume encyclopedia of black athletes from antiquity to the present, lists thousands of standouts. And people of color have received advice about the role of physical activity in weight loss since at least the eleventh century, when an influential Arabian physician by the name of Avicenna prescribed "hard exercise" for overcoming obesity. Like the Greeks before him, Avicenna realized that exercise does something magical for the body. In the thousand years since, doctors have advised us, cajoled us, lectured us, cautioned us, and sometimes even pleaded with us to exercise. But have we listened? Hardly. At any given time, about half of all overweight Americans are trying to lose weight, according to the Centers for Disease Control. But only 25 percent do it through a combination of diet and exercise.

One of the reasons that so many people don't exercise may be a sense of resignation. Given the many health risks of obesity and the difficulty of losing weight, it can be tempting to give up on exercise even before you try it. "Many of us have developed an all-or-nothing attitude," NAAFA board member Nancy Summer told *Ms.* magazine. "If we can't be thin, we may as well not worry about nutrition or exercise—we are going to die young anyway." Summer, who weighs 300 pounds, adds, "I think it's time we reject that concept."

Indeed, there are lots of reasons why exercise can help obese people:

Exercise helps you lose weight. According to one estimate, about 75 percent of the calories we eat go to maintain normal body functions—to fuel our heart and brain, grow new cells, dispose of wastes, and so forth. These calories are essential. The other 25 percent are up for grabs. In active people (including children), the extra calories get burned up when we take a stroll through the park, climb a flight of stairs, wash windows—anything that forces us to use our muscles. In sedentary people, the calories pile up instead of getting burned up. Forging ahead with an exercise regimen can put those calories to good use where they belong—in the body's furnace, not the pantry.

You can lose more weight with exercise and good nutrition than with nutrition alone. Most people—80 percent of all women dieters and 75 percent of all men—try to lose weight by eating less. That's simply not enough. Only by incorporating exercise with a nutritious diet do you have a fighting chance at keeping unwanted pounds at bay. Otherwise, you're fair game for the body's biological drive to replace what you lose.

Need more evidence? In a University of Pittsburgh comparison of black and white women, black women's extra weight could not be explained by diet, because both groups ate the same number of calories. The major behavioral difference was activity level. Black women climbed fewer stairs, walked fewer city blocks, and played fewer sports than their white counterparts did—a finding that prompted investigators to urge black women to exercise more instead of eating less.

Still not convinced? Look at what happened in California, where Stanford researchers pitted diet against exercise in a head-to-head challenge. There were two groups of men. The average weight was 220 pounds. One group went on a diet that reduced their daily intake by 300 calories. The second group got to eat their normal diet, but walked or ran 10 to 12 miles a week. By the end of the first year, the dieters had lost an average of 12 pounds of body fat, and 15 pounds overall. The exercisers lost only 9. But at the end of three years, the dieters had regained all of their lost weight. The exercisers kept theirs off.

If you want the secret to successful long-term weight loss, look no further than the 784 men and women who've enrolled in the National Weight Control Registry, which tracks people who've lost at least 30 pounds and kept it off for at least a year. Although most had been obese since childhood, they registered an average of 66 lost pounds and maintained it over an average of 5½ years. What's their secret? Eighty-eight percent of them had one thing on common, according to researchers at the University of Colorado and the University of Pittsburgh: They continued to diet and exercise once they had achieved their desired weight loss.

Eating well is good. But eating well and exercising is better. "Exercise is the most important part of any weight-loss program," says Dr. Lalita Kaul, a Howard University College of Medicine professor of clinical nutrition. One researcher goes so far as to say that fat people should be considered "underexercised" rather than "overfed."

Exercise doesn't make you eat more. It's understandable to worry that exercising might make you ravenous. Just take a glimpse at an athletic training table, where heavy exercisers chow down mountainous piles of edibles. But when doctors advise fat people to exercise, they're not suggesting flying to Boston to run in the next marathon. What they have in mind is usually much more modest — twenty or thirty minutes of moderate to moderately strenuous activity (even walking qualifies) — performed at least several times a week. This level of activity simply isn't enough to significantly increase most people's appetites.

In fact, if anyone feels hungrier after this sort of exercise, it's likely to be average-weight people. When people of average weight exercise, they typically eat a little more. It's their body's way of compensating for having used up additional calories; the extra food restores an energy balance so that the number of calories coming into the body matches the energy going out. Overweight people don't show that same precise energy balance. Unlike thinner people, fat people don't eat more in response to exercise. That turns out to be a nice benefit for a large person who's trying to lose weight, because it means that you can exercise without fear that your resulting appetite will cause you to wolf down so much food that you'll quickly wipe out your newly established calorie debt.

Exercise helps reverse the dangerous side effects of obesity. Too much body weight causes a number of disturbances in body chemistry. It floods the bloodstream with fats, thus increasing the risk of heart disease. It builds up insulin in the blood and makes the body less sensitive to insulin, both of which are not only the first step down the road to diabetes but can also lead to high blood pressure.

These are all metabolic disturbances that indicate an imbalance in how the body takes in energy (in the form of food) and gives off energy (in the form of heat). Exercise can help correct these imbalances. It makes muscle tissue more responsive to insulin, thereby helping sugars move more normally from the bloodstream to the muscles, which use them for fuel. Correcting this insulin imbalance can alleviate high blood pressure and diabetes. In fact, some diabetics find that with good diet and regular exercise, they no longer need to take insulin. Finally, exercise also clears fats from the bloodstream, thereby guarding against a buildup of fatty arterial deposits that can lead to heart disease, hardening of the arteries, and stroke.

These wonderful benefits last only for a day or two, which is why doctors advise working out at least three times a week. But what you gain far outweighs the cost. At Sweden's University of Göteborg, obesity and exercise expert Dr. Per Björntorp says that the many health benefits of exercising aren't always appreciated. "In the treatment of obesity, these effects of exercise may be considered at least equally as important as a decrease in body weight," he says. "If body fat loss also results from the exercise program, the beneficial effects are even more pronounced."

Of course, weight loss is one of the welcome effects of exercise. Exercising not only speeds up your metabolism so you burn more calories, but it also helps replace fat with muscle. In metabolic terms, that's like replacing a tortoise with a hare; muscle tissue is so much more metabolically active that exercisers often find they lose weight without even changing their diet.

How much weight can you reasonably expect to lose with an exercise program? It depends on so many variables—your body chemistry, your diet, the type of exercise, the frequency of your workouts. One thing's for sure, though: Many African-Americans should think twice before rushing headlong for the ideal weights defined by insurance company tables. Howard University's Dr. Lalita Kaul explains: "When people come into our clinic, I don't even look at the tables. It's simply not realistic for a 300-pound black person to aim for weighing 125 pounds, which is what the insurance companies say she should weigh. We try to encourage more reasonable goals—maybe losing 50 of those 300 pounds and concentrating on maintaining that new weight."

Health experts agree. "The best approach to combating obesity is through physical activity," says U.S. Surgeon General Dr. David Satcher. But don't feel that you have to end up looking like a supermodel, because most people just don't have the genes for it. Instead, 15 percent weight loss is just about ideal for an obese person. For a 200-pound person, that means dropping 30 pounds and keeping them off. If you can do that, you're more of a success story than any supermodel. (After all, anyone can walk down a runway, right?) Obesity experts agree: Focus less on thinness, more on health. "Instead of having the goal of weight loss," University of California at Davis nutrition professor Judith Stern told the *Washington Post,* "the new goal is weight management, which is achieving the best weight possible in the context of overall health."

STARTING AN EXERCISE PROGRAM

Bear in mind that some exercisers lose more weight than others. Fat on the hips, thighs, and buttocks is much harder to lose than abdominal fat. That explains why obese men, whose fat is usually concentrated in a "spare tire," generally find it easier to lose weight than do women, whose fat is centered around the reproductive organs. It also explains why women with apple-type physiques often lose weight more readily than do women whose bodies more resemble a pear.

Overweight people who are contemplating an exercise program should bear in mind a number of considerations:

First, consult a doctor. Anyone, regardless of their weight, who's in their thirties or older and who hasn't exercised in a while should check with a physician before beginning a workout program. For overweight people, it pays to be even more cautious: Regardless of age, you should see a doctor first. A physician can evaluate any extra risk of heart disease and other ailments and either give you the green light to begin or specify conditions under which you can exercise safely. For example, doctors often prescribe exercise for diabetics, because it lowers a person's blood sugar. Diabetics might be counseled to check their blood sugar before and after exercising to make sure that their blood sugar stays in the safe range.

Start slowly. There may be a triathlete inside of you yearning to be free, but it's safer to start your workouts gently. Begin with 5 or so minutes of exercise and add 5 minutes a week until you can stay active for 30 to 60 minutes. In fact, if you're very large, it may be better to simply limber up your body with stretches and strengthening exercises. Over the weeks, once your body is accustomed to the new movements, you can progress to more strenuous exercise.

I recently tried a weight-control plan that included half an hour of daily exercise on a treadmill or exercise bike. With this regime I lost both weight and inches. But the memorable part of the experience for me was how slowly I had to start exercising. I was in such poor physical condition that at first I was winded after 5 minutes. But as I continued, my tolerance for the exercise increased. Soon I found I would walk up stairs more easily, or walk a few city blocks without really noticing it.

Try to be aware of your body's needs. Fat people, particularly those with a history of eating disorders and the stresses that lead to them, sometimes have a dual relationship with their bodies. After learning to disregard or even punish their bodies by eating too much, binging, or other manifestations of eating disorders, heavy people who start exercise programs must learn a new sense of body awareness. "Many overweight people, accustomed to living from the neck up, tend to ignore signals of distress from the lower body," writes *New York Times* health columnist Jane E. Brody. "But, while exercising, it is important to realize that symptoms like breathing difficulties, chest or muscle pain, and weakness are warnings to slow down, modify, or stop the activity."

Normal healthy exercise can leave you winded, and it can cause a certain degree of discomfort. Pain, however, can be a sign of injury. When in doubt, it's good to check with an exercise instructor, a recreational therapist, or your doctor. In time, as you grow increasingly attuned to your body, you will learn to distinguish between mere discomfort and the warning sign of pain.

And don't forget to eat enough to fuel your body. One-half of the weight lost during very low-calorie diets isn't from fat. It's from muscle and bone, and you need to hang on to yours. Plan on eating about 250 fewer calories a day (and burning up 250 more calories) than you did before starting your exercise program. If you're on a weight-loss program that counts points, the point counting will help you eat at

How Strenuous Is Strenuous?

People measure the intensity of exercise by counting heartbeats. Everyone has a maximum heart rate—the fastest your heart will pump under any circumstances, regardless of the demands the body is placing on it. This heart rate (it's called *maximum aerobic capacity,* or *MAC*) declines with age. To find yours, subtract your age from the number 220.

It's too taxing to ask your heart to go all-out, even if you're in peak condition. Anyway, you don't need to push your cardiovascular system that hard to benefit from exercise. If you're just starting an exercise program, aim for 60 to 75 percent of exercising all-out. Take your MAC and multiply it by .60. The result is the lowest pulse rate (per minute) that you should reach during exercise. Now multiply your MAC by .75. This is the highest pulse rate you should reach. (One easy way to measure your pulse during exercise is to record the number of heartbeats for ten seconds and multiply by six.) Once you get accustomed to this level of intensity, you can increase the pace of your workout to the point that your heart rate is 85 percent of your MAC.

Here's an example. A forty-year-old woman wants to start an exercise program. Her maximum aerobic capacity is 220 minus her age, or 180. She multiplies 180 by .60 and .75 to calculate her targeted minimum and maximum heart rates (108 and 135 beats per minute, respectively). Once she feels comfortable at that level of activity, she can gradually increase her workouts to the point where she has a heart rate approaching 85 percent of her MAC, or 153 beats per minute.

the appropriate amount. If your program lets you eat any amount of allowable food, gradually reduce the portion size until you start to lose weight.

Protect your body from undue stresses. Use well-padded shoes on a cushioned surface. Wear comfortable, loose-fitting clothes in a cool, well-ventilated area. Avoid exercises that call for bending at the waist or compressing your chest—two uncomfortable stresses for heavy people.

Find an exercise routine that's right for you. There's a

common misconception that exercise can't be fun. "Exercise should be enjoyable," says Dr. Lalita Kaul of the Howard University Medical School. "I always tell people that if they like to dance, turn on some music and exercise to that. If they like to walk, make a daily routine of walking through the neighborhood, if it's safe. Individualize your program so it suits your needs." Barry Franklin, a heart specialist at William Beaumont Hospital in Royal Oak, Michigan, recommends that aerobic conditioning for fat people be camouflaged as games, relays, and stunts involving balls, hula hoops, jump ropes, parachutes — you name it. This approaches "emphasizes fun, pleasure, and repeated success," says Franklin, "in contrast to the pain and discomfort associated with many traditional and rehabilitative exercise programs." You'll find lots of friendly, supportive advice on designing a complete exercise program in *Great Shape: The First Fitness Guide for Large Women* by Pat Lyons, R.N., and Debby Burgard (Bull Publishing, 1990). See the box below for more ideas.

The most important thing to remember is the

"Heavy" Ideas for Breaking into Exercise

If you're a plus-size person, you may find the idea of starting an exercise regimen—not to mention actually doing it—a real challenge. Here are some resources geared to heavy folks:

- *Radiance: The Magazine for Large Women,* $20 for one-year subscription (four issues) to: P.O. Box 30246, Oakland, CA 94604; (510) 482-0680; Web site: www.radiancemagazine.com
- *Idrea — The Larger Woman's Workout,* 47-minute video, $19.95 plus $4.50 shipping from: Collage Video, (800) 793-0666.

- *Yoga for Round Bodies I & II,* 50-minute video, $19.95 plus $4.50 shipping from: Collage Video, (800) 793-0666.
- *WIN: The Weight Control Information Network,* operated by the National Institute of Diabetes and Digestive and Kidney Diseases, One WIN Way, Bethesda, MD 20892-3662; (800) WIN-8098; Web site: www.niddk.nih.gov/NutritionDocs.html
- The National Coalition for Promoting Physical Activity offers fact sheets and information for new and continuing exercises. P.O. Box 1440, Indianapolis, IN 46206; Web site: www.ncppci.org
- *Shape Up America!,* a not-for-profit coalition of industry, medical/health, nutrition, and physical fitness organizations chaired by former U.S. Surgeon General C. Everett Koop, 6707 Democracy Blvd., Suite 206, Bethesda, MD 20817.
- *American Obesity Association,* a not-for-profit coalition of health professionals and laypersons geared to helping people achieve a healthy weight, P.O. Box 7114, Madison, WI 53707.

right attitude. Not too long ago, the vast majority of obesity experts believed that a fat person who wanted to be healthier had only one alternative. "We had it drummed into our heads that the only route to fitness is through weight loss," explains NAAFA board member Nancy Summer. Today, more and more people are realizing just the opposite—that the only route to weight loss is through fitness. And indeed, that weight loss isn't even the primary goal anymore. The goal is to feel good about ourselves. You might begin exercising be-

How to Find Like Minds (and Bodies) for Exercise

Lots of exercise outlets around the country cater to heavy people. Many YMCAs, hospitals, and health clubs offer programs that include low-impact aerobics or dance-exercise classes. Water aerobics, which are exceptionally gentle on the body, are particularly useful for people with very large bodies.

cause you want to lose weight, but what keeps you going is a new calm that envelops you, a heightened sense of self-esteem, a deep relaxation that brings quiet joy to everyday life. Once that happens, lots of other benefits are apt to come tumbling our way.

CHAPTER 6

If Dieting Doesn't Work, What Should I Eat?

Black people have a special relationship with food. We may not always have much money, but we invariably celebrate weddings and graduations and reunions with the most generous platters that we can afford. Many of us observe Kwanzaa, an African celebration of the harvest, which has taken its place alongside other holidays on the African-American calendar. Even when someone dies, the neighbors and friends who visit the survivors may come grieving, but they also come with casseroles and roasts and foil-covered pies.

Why do African-Americans have such a strong connection with food? Perhaps it's our recent experience of not having very much of it. Not too long ago, our slave forebears subsisted on what sometimes amounted to very little nourishment indeed. Each Saturday night, slaves would receive their weekly allotment of a peck and a half of cornmeal and three pounds of bacon. Sometimes this meager diet was supplemented with fish, vegetables, or molasses. Slaves rarely starved to death; an owner had too strong a stake in keeping his investment alive. But investments are also designed to turn a profit, and for that reason slaves were fed as cheaply as possible. Historian Richard Sutch calls the typical slave diet "monotonous, crude, and nutritionally suspect."

Now fast-forward to the present. Food has become so plentiful that African-Americans are actually *dieting*. Every new diet book that comes along finds its way into eager brown hands. Black women sit under beauty parlor hair dryers discussing their latest forays in weight management; black men, mindful of their girth, think twice about reaching for that second slab of pie—a luxury practically unheard of a century and a half ago. Hunger in America has by no means disappeared, but millions of African-Americans no longer struggle to get enough to eat. If anything, the struggle is the exact reverse: to refrain from eating too much.

How did we get from there to here? Credit modern agriculture for much of the change. Over the years, the American food supply grew increasingly abundant, and our food transportation system began to allow a family in Fort Wayne, Indiana, to sample California cabbage, Florida flounder, and Texas T-bones. In addition to this sudden cornucopia, black families continued to enjoy the foods we had grown accustomed to during slavery—foods that we loved but that weren't always paragons of nutrition. As black nutritionist Josephine Schuyler warned during World War II, "Of all Americans, Negroes most need to know about food. They have the worst health and the worst eating habits in the country."

Somewhere along the line, African-Americans started to cross over from having too little food to having a bit too much. Black doctors and nutritionists began to warn us about the dangers of excess weight. "For those who wish to lose cumbersome pounds, now is the time!" suggested Tuskegee Institute's *Service* magazine in 1952. "Proper weight is extremely important to an individual's general health," advised a 1950 health column in the NAACP's *The Crisis* magazine. "It is not difficult to plan a diet that will lead to loss of weight."

Well, to plan a diet you must first select one. And on that score, we have shown an ingenuity and originality that is distinctly African-American. Bear in mind that in the early 1950s black doctors were dispensing the same recommendations that many health professionals give today: Cut down on sugars and fats, try smaller portions, and eat plenty of whole grains and nutrient-rich vegetables. In the face of this advice, prominent African-Americans (and presumably many others) followed their own instincts. *Their* prescriptions appeared in the black press, often accompanied by personal testimonies.

Trumpeter Louis Armstrong started the ball rolling in 1956 with an unusual regimen that he termed the "Satchmo Diet." "For breakfast, you have a large glass of orange juice and black coffee or tea," the legendary jazzman told *Ebony*. "For lunch, you have anything you want but just have tomatoes with lemon juice over it. Then at suppertime eat anything from soup to nuts, but you should have greens, which are good for the stomach." Armstrong's unusual prescription was more than good for his stomach, he said; the trumpeter lost 98 pounds in a few months. He was so pleased that he wrote another dieter — President Eisenhower. "I told the president to do it the Satchmo way and he'd feel ten years old," Armstrong recalled, smiling. "He wrote back and said as president he isn't supposed to feel like he's ten years old."

In the 1970s, *Ebony* presented more celebrity diets. Singer Johnny Mathis swore off bread and fats, dug into fruits and vegetables, and prepared many of his own meals. "When I'm working, I usually eat only one meal a day—something very nourishing but not fattening," said Mathis, looking fit. "It has taken me many years of traveling around the world and visiting exotic places to learn that many people actually do dig their graves with their forks."

Barry White used the one-meal-a-day trick, too. The singer simply grew tired of devouring whole fried chickens and quarts of ice cream. At 360 pounds, White stood naked before a mirror and cursed himself for traveling the world singing about love when he didn't love himself enough to slim down. So it was one meal a day—Chinese food every afternoon at 2:00 P.M. "Why Chinese food? Because it's light and not so fattening and doesn't stay on your stomach very long," he told *Jet*. After thus breaking his habit of eating all day long, White moved on to even stronger medicine. He would prepare a plate of food, look at it, nibble it, smell it. "Just enough to satisfy my tastebuds. Then I'd dump it in the garbage can. The willpower I'd built up had told me 'O.K. now, Barry, don't eat that stuff. Remember, you're the one who's got the most to lose.'" One hundred pounds, in fact, which he lost over the course of a year.

In 1974, actress Jayne Kennedy revealed a diet that she said worked well for her. "You can eat a lot of meat and you get all your vitamins but no carbohydrates at all." Dancer Eartha Kitt added to the confusion when she told *Ebony*, "I don't think milk is good for you either, although if you do drink three glasses of milk a day, it cleans out the whole body. But the Danish doctors say that the kind of fat that comes from milk and other cow products is hardest to get rid of."

These represent just a few of the probably thousands of diets that black Americans have tried over the years. Some diets may work, at least for a while; others may be useless or even ill-advised. Satchmo's morning orange juice would be disastrous for diabetics, who must restrict the intake of sugars; Jayne Kennedy's meat-centered diet could strain the kidneys, which help the body handle protein digestion. And while the one-meal-a-day plan might be reasonable for an elderly person whose calorie needs are very modest, the same regimen would be foolhardy for a growing teenager and even dangerous for a pregnant or breast-feeding woman, who needs extra helpings of calories.

Indeed, nutritionists warn us that a fair number of the many popular diet plans on the market at any one time are questionable. They either provide too few calories or too much or too little of a certain nutrient, or they're prohibitively expensive, or they don't call for all-important exercise. Some can present health hazards. Dr. Johanna Dwyer, professor of medicine and community health at Tufts University Medical School, has drawn up a list of nutritional criteria for judging the value of some diet plans that have been popular in the last decade or so. Based on these criteria, most of the diets—42 of 60—fall short.

The National Institutes of Health minces no words about diet plans. A 1992 NIH conference of weight-loss experts emerged with this stark warning: "The panel cautions that before individuals adopt any program for the purpose of losing weight, they should examine the scientific data available documenting their safety and efficacy. If no such data exist, the panel recommends that the program not be utilized." Since few popular diet plans have been rigorously tested for safety and effectiveness, NIH's advice essentially shuts the door on most of them.

What, then, are the best options for someone interested in a sound eating program? Well, you can join a supervised weight-loss program at a clinic, hospital, or

Criteria Consumers Can Use in Judging Popular Diet Plans

1. Is the program safe? Is there medical supervision or are periodic physical checks by physicians required?
2. Does the plan include aerobic and other physical activity and exercise?
3. Is the rate of weight loss reasonable (4 to 8 pounds per month)?
4. Is the diet too restrictive?
5. Is the diet nutritionally balanced?
6. Does the diet use liquid formulas rather than foods, and if so, are suitable precautions taken and is the formula nutritionally adequate?
7. Does the program prescribe appetite suppressants of unproven efficacy?
8. Can the diet be followed?
9. Does the program make scientific and common sense?
10. Does it suit the dieter's particular psychological, social, and physiological needs? Does it deal with emotional adjustments to weight loss? Does it include behavioral and environmental modification techniques?
11. Are individual or group motivation and support provided to help the dieter assume responsibility for weight loss?
12. Is the cost reasonable? Are special foods, special devices, books, or fees required?
13. Will provision be made for weight maintenance and keeping weight off after the program ends?
14. Does the diet permit the dieter to monitor the program?

Recommendations reproduced by permission of Dr. Johanna Dwyer, the Frances Stern Nutrition Center of the New England Medical Center Hospitals. From Dwyer JT. Treatment of obesity. In: Bjorntorp P., Brodoff B. *Obesity*. Philadelphia: Lippincott, 1992:664,668.

Some Reasonable and Questionable Diets for the Treatment of Obesity

1,200 calories per day or more

Reasonable diets
I Don't Eat (But I Can't Lose) Weight Control Program
Harvard Square Diet
Red Book Wise Women's Diet
Doctor's Calorie Plus
Behavioral Control Diet
California Nutrition Book
California Diet
LEARN Program for Weight Control Complete University Medical Diet

Questionable diets
Oat and Wheat Bran Health Plan
New Canadian Fiber Diet (DePrey)
Women's Advantage Diet (Mallek)
The 35 Plus Diet for Women
Bad Back Diet Book (Green and Ceresa)
"T" Factor Diet
The Mediterranean Diet
Atkin's Diet Revolution
Nutrition Breakthrough
Dr. Abravanel's Body Type Diet
Doctor's Quick Weight Loss
Pritikin Program Diet
Craig Claibourne's Gourmet Diet
Rechtschaffen Diet
Orthocarbohydrate Diet
Easy No Risk Diet
Slender Now
Never Say Diet
F Plan Diet
Carbohydrate Craver's Diet
Dr. Atkin's Health Revolution
Immune Power
What Your Doctor Didn't Learn in Medical School

800 to 1,199 calories per day

Reasonable diets
Lean and Green Diet
Hilton Head Metabolism Diet
Weight Watcher's Quick Start
Diet Workshop Lo Carbo and Beacon Hill Diets

Questionable diets
Two Day Diet
Rotation Diet
Diet Workshop Wild Weekend
The Hilton Head Over 35 Diet
L.A. Diet
Doctor's Metabolic Diet
No Choice Diet
Woman Doctor's Diet
Southhampton Diet
Bloomingdale Diet
Snowbird Diet
Herbalife Slim Trim Diet
Fit for Life
Thin So Fast (Eades)
The Rice Diet
Beverly Hills Diet

800 calories or less

Reasonable diets (only if administered under medical supervision)
HMR (Health Management Resources)
Optifast
United Weight Control
New Directions (Ross Labs)
Nutrisystem

Questionable diets
Herbalife
Last Chance Diet
Fasting Is a Way of Life

Recommendations reproduced by permission of Dr. Johanna Dwyer, the Frances Stern Nutrition Center of the New England Medical Center Hospitals. From Dwyer JT. Treatment of obesity. In: Bjorntorp P., Brodoff B. *Obesity*. Philadelphia: Lippincott, 1992:664,668.

How to Evaluate a Supervised Weight-Loss Program

Here are the twelve most important questions to ask about any commercial, hospital-based, or clinic-based weight-loss program, according to the National Institutes of Health:

1. How many people who start the program finish it? The dropout rates for some programs range as high as 80 percent. Two in ten odds aren't very high.
2. How many people who finish the program achieve various degrees of weight loss?
3. How much of that weight loss is maintained after one, three, or even five years?
4. How many participants experience negative side effects from the program?
5. What's the nature of the side effects, and how severe are they?
6. What mix of diet, exercise, and behavior modification does the program call for? The best programs include all three.
7. How much counseling is included, and what type is it? Individual or closed-group counseling is more effective than open groups in which members are free to come and go.
8. How many disciplines does the staff represent? The most effective programs involve a range of experts: physicians, nutritionists, psychologists, physiologists, etc.
9. Does the program prepare you to prevent relapses that can occur in stressful situations?
10. How long is the maintenance phase of the program, and what does it consist of?
11. How flexible are your food choices?
12. Are weight goals set by the program or in cooperation with participants? The more input participants have, the more they are likely to stick with the program and benefit from it.

commercial outlet. Or you can develop your own plan that you can live with—one that reflects your personality and the types of food that you like to eat. You may find that assembling your own dietary plan gives you a sense of ownership and pride that helps you stick with the program. That's what the remainder of this chapter is devoted to. Either way you go—whether with a packaged diet plan or your own—we will assume that you are already committed to an exercise program. (Are you?)

CONSTRUCTING YOUR PERSONAL EATING PLAN

Think about the word *diet* for a moment. Almost any diet will help you lose weight, at least for a while. But the problem is that if you are "on" a diet, you can be "off" one, too. All it takes is a little temptation, a few seconds of weakness. Our favorite food sneaks up on us, and before we know it, it bushwacks us in plain daylight. "Everybody's had those moments when you thought you were in control and then just lost it," Oprah Winfrey told her studio audience. "And then something happens in your brain…You don't know what it is. You find yourself in the refrigerator attached to it." And then once we're off a diet, it becomes that much easier to rationalize going off it again whenever temptation might strike. We feel guiltier and guiltier, we get fatter and fatter, and the entire counterproductive exercise does a crash and burn.

So let's not use the word *diet.* Instead, consider this a plan to renovate your usual food choices. The emphasis will be on assembling a dietary strategy. In a sense, you will actually reteach yourself how to enjoy eating. And when you finish this chapter, you will want to eat to live instead of wanting to live to eat.

Let's start with a basic overview of what's in food. This will allow you to select the foods that are the best for both taste and health. Below we'll review the six basic nutrients that the body needs in order to function.

These are water, carbohydrates, proteins, fats, vitamins, and minerals. All nutrients must come from our diet.

Everyone has heard of calories. These are the sources of energy or fuel that the body uses to run our basic life-support systems. Calories keep our heart beating, our lungs breathing, our digestive tract absorbing food, and so forth. Calories come from carbohydrates, proteins, and fats.

Water

A renowned biologist once described people as the "way that water has of going about beyond the reach of rivers." You and I are 85 percent water, and everything that happens inside of us, every process that keeps us alive, depends on water. Water makes up most of the eight quarts of blood that circulate throughout the body. Water is what dissolves nutrients so they can be carried by the blood. Water is what waste products dissolve into so they can be flushed from our system. In terms of day-to-day survival, water is our most important nutrient.

Water is found in all fruits, vegetables, milk products, meats, poultry, and fish. Breads, cereals, nuts, and dried beans contain much less water. Doctors recommend that we consume eight glasses of water—two quarts—each day for normal fluid balance. Because our food contains so much water, most of us actually eat about half of the water that we take in. The other half comes from beverages. If you're not sure whether you're getting enough water, the best indicator is the body's signal: thirst.

There's nothing wrong with keeping your body primed with water. Water helps flush the kidneys and helps prevent kidney stones and urinary tract infections. In fact, if you're trying to lose weight, drinking extra water is a very good idea indeed. Some low-calorie diets cause the body to break down proteins, which then need to be flushed out of your system; drinking lots of water helps ensure that your body has enough fluid to do the job. A glass of water before or with meals may also help calm hunger signals.

In simpler times, water was water. Nowadays we have so many more choices—mineral water, flavored water, sparkling water. Tap water is all your body needs to be healthy. However, if your doctor has advised you to watch your sodium intake, you should know that some municipal water supplies and some bottled water can be high in sodium. A water softener in your home can also increase sodium levels. If your tap water contains more than 20 milligrams of sodium per quart, you might consider switching to bottled water. Your local health department can advise you on how to have your water tested for sodium and other minerals.

If straight water is unappealing to you, consider a twist of lemon, lime, or grapefruit rind to give it a citrus essence. Or try any of a variety of caffeine-free hot or cold teas. But steer clear of teas or other beverages

How to Recognize Ingredients That Cause Water Loss

You might spot these on the label of an herbal tea, another beverage, or a food. They aren't harmful to your health, but if you're trying to keep your body hydrated, you may want to avoid them.

Diuretics (cause increased urine output):

Caffeine, cranberry juice, watermelon or watermelon seeds, or the following herbs: bearberry, broom tops, buchu, burdock, cleavers, couch grass, hydrangea, juniper, parsley, parsley piert, pellitory-of-the-wall, queen of the meadow, stinging nettle, stone root, wild carrot, yarrow.

Laxatives (cause gentle bowel stimulation):

Cascara, castor oil plant, chia seed, flaxseed, licorice, olive oil, psyllium, rhubarb, senna.

Cathartics (cause complete bowel evacuation):

Black root, butternut, castor oil plant, jalapa, May-apple or American mandrake, mountain flax, rhubarb, senna.

that contain diuretics—ingredients that increase the flow of urine. Caffeine is a diuretic. So is alcohol. (That's why it doesn't make sense to drink beer to quench your thirst on a hot day; the alcohol simply causes you to lose more fluid than you take in.) Also take care to avoid herbal teas that contain laxatives or cathartics. These stimulate bowel movements, which cause water loss.

Carbohydrates

Carbohydrates are sugars and starches. You get 4 calories in a gram of carbohydrate. In their simplest form—sugars—carbohydrates are found as a natural ingredient in a variety of foods, including fruits, fruit juices, honey, fresh sugar cane, and molasses. Sugar may also be refined from sugar cane and sugar beets (as in granulated sugar) and added to foods ranging from soft drinks and desserts to candy. Whether the sugar is refined or not, the body recognizes all simple carbohydrates as sugar. To the tongue, their sweetness is immediately evident and pleasurable.

Starches—complex carbohydrates—are simply sugars that are linked together into complex arrangements. One way to visualize the difference between simple and complex sugars is to picture a tree. The simple sugars are represented by the leaves, which are attached to the many branches. The entire tree, with its complex arrangement of leaves, represents a starch.

Some sugars and starches are made with the same basic raw ingredient: a sugar called glucose. You don't taste the glucose in a cracker or a piece of bread. But if you chew it for a while, you might detect a faint sweetness. That's the

Carbohydrates in Our Diet

Type	Name	Found in foods such as...
Simple	Glucose, fructose, and sucrose	Fruits, juices, syrup, table sugar; small amounts in vegetables; soft drinks and desserts
	Lactose	Milk, yogurt, cheese
	Dextrose	Small amounts in fruits and vegetables; also added to foods in small amounts
Complex	Starch	Beans, peas, wheat, rice, oatmeal, corn, barley, root vegetables (potatoes, yams, turnips, carrots), plantains, and any foods made from these foods (such as bread, rice cakes, crackers, spaghetti, cereals)
Fiber	Cellulose, pectin, gum	Found throughout foods that come from plants, including fruits and vegetables, and in the bran of wheat, rice, oats, corn, beans, and peas.

Choosing High-Fiber Alternatives

Low Fiber Instead of refined grains...	**High Fiber** Have whole grains...
White flour	Whole wheat flour
White bread	Whole wheat bread
White rice	Brown rice
Degerminated corn meal	Stone-ground corn meal
Fruit or vegetable juice	Whole fruit or vegetable
Peeled apple or potato	Apple or potato with skin
Simple lettuce salad	Lettuce salad with lots of extras: cucumbers, beans, celery, etc.

glucose, after an enzyme in your saliva has had a chance to break down the starch into sugar.

There's one additional kind of carbohydrate: fiber, also called roughage. Fiber is found in fruits, vegetables, and whole grains. It's mostly cellulose, the same tough material found in grass and wood. Ruminant animals, like cows, host bacteria in their stomachs that produce special enzymes to break down cellulose and make the glucose available for calories. Humans can't, which is why fiber passes through our digestive tract intact. However, fiber serves a valuable purpose by cleansing the intestines and preventing constipation.

As a rule, all carbohydrates—whether sugars, starches, or fiber—play an important role in our health. But we are a nation of sugar-holics. We eat so much sugar that it often takes up too much of a day's allotment of calories. When a food is practically all sugar with no vitamins, minerals, or protein, it's called a source of "empty" or "hollow" calories. It's a source of calories, but little else of the nutrients that we need for good health.

To enjoy the natural goodness of carbohydrates, aim for high-fiber foods. These include whole grains, which contain the bran and the germ. Modern food processors like to strip away these important parts of the grain because the bulky bran makes for a less uniform flour, and the oil-rich germ can go rancid if not refrigerated. But what's convenient for the food packagers is deadly for us food consumers. Not enough fiber can contribute to a number of digestive disorders, including constipation, hemorrhoids, and possibly colon cancer.

Fat

Fat is the densest source of calories in our diet. Each gram supplies 9 calories. In other words, gram for gram, fat provides over twice as many calories as carbohydrates (at 4 calories per gram). If you eat too much fat, you'll put on pounds twice as quickly as you will if you eat too many carbohydrates.

Fat is one of those nutrients that we love and hate. On the one hand, it gives foods thickness, creaminess, and richness. It delays emptying of the stomach, so a meal lasts longer before you feel hungry again. We need fat to help us absorb so-called fat-soluble vitamins—A, D, E, and K. It is also needed for certain life-sustaining functions.

But too much fat is bad news. Overconsumption of fat has been linked to high cholesterol levels, hypertension, stroke, diabetes, cancer, and a condition that worsens all of these health problems—obesity.

Many African-Americans learned to use fat to prepare Southern food. In an earlier era, we needed generous amounts of fats to fill in for more nutritious foods that were unavailable. When scarcity was the norm and not the exception, our people made the best of what they had; we used whatever food ingredients that were inexpensive and that filled our stomachs. At a time when a slave's inability to work the fields could mean severe reprisals, fats were precious: meat drippings were saved, butter was skimmed from milk, lard was rendered. Pork skins, which are almost all fat, were turned into side dishes. Limited cooking facilities meant that most slave families cooked in a single pot, often relying on a single cooking method: frying. Everything was fried—hush puppies, potatoes, eggs. In good times, there was fried chicken and fried fish. More often, whatever meat came into the home was dictated by a slaveowner's discarded scraps: pork rinds, pigs' feet, ham hocks, chitterlings, all low in protein and high in fat. (The fact that slaveowners enjoyed the choicest cuts of pork—ham, bacon, sausage—gave rise to the term "eating high on the hog.")

Now that we no longer have to depend on fat for our survival, it is time to unlearn our love of fat. It's not easy. When football star William "Refrigerator" Perry ballooned up to 360 pounds and was ordered by his coach to lose some weight, one Chicago weight-loss expert admitted, "Not everyone is born eating like a yuppie. Eating food with high fat content is a hard pattern to break, and despite what nutritionists say we should do, all of us eat when we're not hungry."

But you can start by using less fat, by buying reduced-fat versions of your favorite foods, and by making simple substitutions for fat.

Trimming the Fat from Your Plate

Instead of...	Use...
Fried foods	Baked, broiled, or steamed foods
Sour cream or mayonnaise	Yogurt or reduced-fat sour cream or mayonnaise
Evaporated whole milk	Evaporated skim milk
Whole-milk cottage cheese	Low-fat cottage cheese
Whole-milk mozzarella cheese	Part-skim mozzarella
Melted butter	Dehydrated butter flakes
Butter or margarine in grits	Grated Parmesan cheese
Butter or margarine on bread	Jelly or preserves
Regular crackers	Fat-free crackers
Whole eggs	Egg whites
Fatty meat	Lean meat with fat trimmed
Chicken (dark meat)	Chicken (white meat)
Tuna packed in oil	Tuna packed in water
Ice cream	Frozen yogurt, ice milk, sherbet

Is Soul Food Good for You?

What's low in fiber, calcium, and potassium, and high in fat, salt, and cholesterol? The answer is soul food, says Dr. Shiriki Kumanyika, a Pennsylvania State University researcher who has studied eating patterns among African-Americans. When Kumanyika surveyed typical black American diets, she found exactly the opposite of what doctors recommend—that is, a diet high in fiber, calcium, and potassium, and low in fat, salt, cholesterol. Clearly a major reason for the sky-high disease rates in our community is the food that we eat.

Fortunately, a little imagination can improve virtually any diet, and soul food is no exception. If you like to cook and bake, one of the easiest ways to cut down on fat and salt is to modify your recipes:

- Try cutting half of the shortening from your homemade biscuits, or use half the salt in your next pot of gumbo. You'd be amazed at how few people will tell the difference.

- To season greens or cabbage without overdosing on grease, try simmering them in canned chicken broth or smoked turkey necks or wings, both of which have little fat. Or boil two ham hocks in water the day before, then cool the broth in the refrigerator and skim off the fat the next day. Then drop in the greens and simmer as usual.
- Baking instead of frying fish or chicken is an obvious fat saver. And when you do use fat, try to substitute polyunsaturated fats like vegetable oil and reduced-calorie spreads for saturated fats like butter and lard. It will help lower your cholesterol.
- Instead of salt, have you ever tried seasoning a creole stew with lemon or lime juice, or black-eyed peas with vinegar? If not, you've missed a treat.
- Try reduced-sodium salt. One brand, Salt Sense® by Akzo Salt Co. of Clarks Summit, Pennsylvania, has 33 percent less sodium and tastes like a dead ringer for the real thing.
- Virtually any vegetable or fruit makes a fine contribution to your fiber intake. And don't forget substitutions like brown rice for white rice and whole wheat rolls for white flour biscuits. These add bran—a great source of fiber—to your diet. Have you ever tried cornbread made with whole wheat flour and stone-ground corn meal? Its full flavor may surprise you.
- If you find that modifying certain dishes takes the "soul" out of them, compromise by serving them less often. Growing numbers of African-Americans reserve their full soul-food spread for holidays and other special occasions instead of daily or weekly fare.

Protein

Protein is a key nutrient. Without protein in our diets, our bodies would have no way to manufacture the cells that make up our skin, muscle, blood, or hair. We'd have no enzymes to digest our food, no hormones to regulate the activity of our many organs. All of these activities take place with the help of amino acids, and amino acids are the stuff of which protein is made.

There are two basic kinds of protein—complete and incomplete. Proteins from animal foods such as milk and meat (but with the exception of gelatin) are complete proteins. Proteins from plant foods such as grains, beans, and vegetables don't supply a complete set of essential amino acids, and are incomplete by themselves. You can get a full set, however, by mixing beans, peas, or legumes with a grain. If you've ever wondered why beans and rice is such a universal dish, the answer is that it contains a perfectly balanced set of amino acids. For that matter, a peanut butter sandwich has the same combination (a legume and wheat). In Mexico, people have thrived for centuries despite eating very little meat. They do it by combining corn and beans, which together supply all of the amino acids they need. Remember the two ways to get high-quality protein:

Animal protein: fish, poultry, lean red meat, eggs, low-fat or nonfat milk, yogurt, low-fat cheese

or

Plant protein: beans, peas, peanuts *with* rice, wheat (bread, cereal, spaghetti, crackers, etc.), corn, oatmeal, barley, etc.

The beans, peas, or legumes can be consumed hours apart from the grain for the two proteins to combine properly.

You may have heard of diets that urge you to eat lots of protein. They go by various names: the Scarsdale Diet, the Calories Don't Count Diet, the Stillman Diet, the Doctor's Quick Weight Loss Diet. The idea is for you to lay off carbohydrates entirely, but to consume all of the chicken, fish, beef, and pork that you want. Proponents of these low-carbohydrate, high-protein diets claim that the technique will elevate your mood and help you protect your health by stimulating weight loss. In actuality, none of the diets work. There's no mood change, except among the people who get rich selling the diet. And because the protein-rich meats and cheeses that people substitute for carbohydrates are often high in fat, the diet may contribute to heart disease. If high-protein diets are so effective, why have millions of people who tried them regained all the weight they initially lost?

The lesson here is simple: Plan a variety of foods that you can live with. We'll return to this important lesson in a few moments.

Vitamins and Minerals

Our bodies need over a dozen vitamins and minerals for life. None are particularly important for weight reduction; vitamin B_6 doesn't help pull fat from fat cells, nor will iodine speed up your thyroid to help you burn calories faster. But if you're watching what you eat and your daily intake falls below 1,500 calories, you may not get all the vitamins and minerals that you need from food. To close any gap, take a low-dose multivitamin. Read the label on the bottle to determine how many milligrams or micrograms of the nutrients are in each pill. The amount should be no more than 100 to 150 percent of the Recommended Dietary Allowances (RDAs).

SETTING WEIGHT GOALS

As we mentioned in Chapter 1, there is no magical number of pounds that you "should" weigh. Some folks consult with a trusted health care professional for an opinion on a reasonable target weight. If you're the type of person who needs concrete numerical goals, this may be the best approach for you. But many find a certain peace of mind in simply aiming

Vitamins and Minerals to Keep Us Strong

NUTRIENT	SOURCES
VITAMIN A	
Helps keep skin smooth and soft. Helps vision; protects against night blindness. Helps keep mucous membranes (lining) of mouth, nose, throat and digestive tract healthy and resistant to infection. Promotes growth.	Dark green and deep yellow vegetables, apricots, cantaloupe, butter, fortified margarine, whole milk, vitamin A-fortified skim milk, cheddar cheese, liver, kidney, eggs
B VITAMINS	
B_1 (Thiamin)	
Needed for proper function of heart and nervous system. Helps obtain energy from food.	Lean meats, fish, poultry, liver, milk, pork, dried yeast, whole-grain cereals, enriched breads and cereals
B_2 (Riboflavin)	
Needed for healthy skin. Helps prevent sensitivity of eyes to light. Needed to build and maintain body tissues.	Eggs, enriched breads and cereals, leafy green vegetables, liver, lean meats, dried yeast, milk
B_6	
Important for healthy gums and teeth and for health of blood vessels, red blood cells, and nervous system.	Wheat germ, vegetables, dried yeast, meats, whole-grain cereals
B_{12}	
Helps prevent certain forms of anemia. Contributes to health of nervous system and to proper growth in children.	Liver, kidney, milk, saltwater fish, oysters, lean meats

Folic Acid	
Helps prevent certain forms of anemia. Needed for health of intestinal tract.	Leafy green vegetables, food yeast, meats
Niacin	
Helps convert food to energy. Aids nervous system and helps prevent loss of appetite.	Lean meats, liver, dried yeast, enriched breads and cereals, eggs
VITAMIN C (Ascorbic Acid)	
Makes intercellular cement that holds body cells together. Strengthens blood vessel walls. Helps resist infection. Helps in more rapid healing of wounds.	Citrus fruits, berries, cantaloupe, broccoli, green and sweet red peppers, tomatoes, raw cabbage, brussels sprouts, potatoes cooked in their skins
VITAMIN D	
Helps body absorb calcium and phosphorous to build strong bones and teeth.	Fish liver oils, vitamin D-fortified milk, egg yolks, salmon, tuna
VITAMIN E	
Acts as an antioxidant to preserve fat-soluble vitamins. Believed necessary for reproduction. May have many other functions; it is still under study.	Vegetable oils, whole-grain cereals, wheat germ, lettuce
VITAMIN K	
Needed for the production of prothrombin, which aids in the normal clotting of blood.	Pork, liver, cabbage, cauliflower, spinach, soybeans
CALCIUM	
Builds bones and teeth. Helps blood to clot. Helps muscles,	Milk (all types), cheese, ice cream, green leafy vegetables

nerves, and heart function properly.	(collards, kale, mustard and turnip greens, broccoli)
IRON	
Combines with protein to make hemoglobin, the red substance in the blood that carries oxygen to all the body cells. Helps cells use oxygen and develop energy.	Lean meats, liver, heart, oysters, dark green leafy vegetables, dried fruits, whole grain and enriched breads and cereals, molasses
IODINE	
Helps thyroid gland function properly by manufacturing the hormone thyroxine that regulates metabolism.	Saltwater fish, shellfish, iodized salt

for a good, balanced diet that's modest in calories. That way, you can stay aware of your weight as you work yourself to better health—but your health, not your weight, stays uppermost.

Either way, it may be helpful to know a few numbers. As we've mentioned, the body stores calories that it doesn't need immediately, and it stores them as fat. As it turns out, it takes 3,500 calories to equal a pound of fat. So if you cut 500 hundred calories a day from your diet, you should lose about a pound at the end of a week, which is the safe, gradual pace that doctors and nutritionists recommend. (If you don't exercise, this weight loss would probably not continue indefinitely, because at some point your metabolism would start to slow down and you would burn fewer calories than before.) It may be difficult to estimate your current intake, but chances are it's greater than 2,000 calories a day. So a 500-calorie deficit should be both sufficient and relatively painless. The menus in Chapter 8 are for a daily intake of 1,500 calories.

How to Set Your Weight-Loss Goals

If you're wondering how much weight is reasonable for you to try to lose, here's what the National Institutes of Health recommend:

- Consider your weight history and the outcomes of past weight-loss efforts. If you have a history of failed diets, are you planning a different strategy this time?
- Consider how much your relatives weigh. Body weight is often inherited, and it may be difficult to get around your genes.
- Think about your emotional profile. Significant, permanent weight loss, when it occurs, takes time and patience. Do you have these?
- Consider logistics. When will you fit your exercise sessions into your day? How will you integrate an eating/exercise plan into a family setting?
- Remember that for most people, achieving the body weight and shape presented in the mass media is neither appropriate nor achievable. So failure to achieve this sort of weight loss doesn't mean you don't have willpower, and it doesn't mean you're somehow deficient in character.
- No matter how much weight you want to lose, remember that it will probably all return within one to five years unless you make permanent changes to your lifestyle by eating wisely and exercising regularly.

WHAT IS YOUR RELATIONSHIP WITH FOOD?

There are lots of biological reasons why people get fat, and there are certainly biological reasons why it is difficult to lose weight. But for many people body weight is tied to their relationship with food. Do you ever eat at night or when you're not hungry? Do you find yourself craving sugar or starch? Do you eat more when you're alone than when you have company? Have you ever caught yourself eating large portions of food because it's there? Is it hard for you to leave food on your plate? Do you eat out a lot?

In a sense, the question here is, do you *eat to live* or *live to eat?* If you live to eat, your food choices are probably guided by a few distinctive rules. See if any of these ring a bell:

- Just about all food tastes good.
- You only live once.
- We're all going to die of something someday, so why not enjoy life?
- Life is rough sometimes, so why deprive myself of a sure pleasure?

If these thoughts lead you by the hand to the nearest refrigerator, you may soon find yourself eating without regard for or despite the nutritional merits of what you're putting in your mouth. Don't get the wrong idea. It's okay to have treats. A "must have" candy bar is not the end of the world. The time to assess whether or not you live to eat is while you are opening the *second* candy bar, or when you are forcing down a too-big portion of peach cobbler immediately after a too-much-on-your-plate dinner, or when you hand the cashier a dollar for a package of gooey cupcakes when less expensive fresh fruit is right there under your nose.

On the other hand, if you eat to live, you may subscribe to a different set of rules:

- Life is precious.
- Health is priceless.

- I *am* in charge of my life.
- I control the forces that bombard me daily.
- Care of my body and soul is of great, nonnegotiable importance.
- I am what I eat.

With this frame of mind, it's easier to appreciate quality foods and make food choices accordingly.

If you find that you lean more toward living to eat, open your mind and soul to change. Start by keeping a food diary. People who have unhealthy relationships with food often eat when they're not even aware of it. The best way to see your food choices for what they really are is to keep track of what you eat, how much you eat, and when you eat. It'll help you identify eating patterns that you may not be aware of.

Use a small notebook. Record what you eat and drink as soon as possible after consuming it. Try to be as thorough and careful with your food diary as you can. Try this format:

Day/Date ______

Time	Food/Amount	Location	Mood	How Hungry

Do your best to know what you are eating and how much you are eating. Here's your list of tools:

- Standard teaspoon: for measuring sugar, butter, margarine
- Standard tablespoon: for measuring salad dressing, mayonnaise, peanut butter

- Standard measuring cup: for measuring rice and cereals
- Food scale: for cheese, meats, fish, chicken, and unsliced breads

Use food labels to help you estimate food quantities. For example, one-half of a 6¼ ounce can of tuna will be approximately 3 ounces of tuna. There's no need to put it on the scale.

The next step is to study your eating habits and plan a strategy.

When Do You Eat?

Look at when you eat a meal or a snack. Are the times that you eat mostly in the evening, after 8:00 P.M.? If so, spread them out over the day. Do you eat late at night, then skip breakfast in the morning? If so, gradually eat your last meal of the day earlier, and eat breakfast the next day earlier as well. Do you let long stretches of time (more than five hours) pass without eating? If so, keep a snack to enjoy somewhere around three hours after a meal. That way, you can stop hunger from taking control of you. Do you eat nonstop? If so, cluster your chain eating into small meals.

The Virtue of Small Meals

Julia Child, the celebrated French chef, doesn't have much patience for nutrition. "What I've seen is a whole lot of nonsense," the venerable kitchen artist told the *Boston Globe,* in reference to current advice to watch what we eat. Child says the problem isn't what we eat but how much we eat. "You don't see many fat people in France, because they eat smaller portions," she said. "If I ate all I wanted, I'd be Mrs. Six-by-Six. What makes sense is to have everything in moderation. People can have steak, but smaller portions."

> Science could prove Julia Child correct. When you eat large meals, your body sends out a burst of insulin. That helps transport glucose (sugar) from your digestive tract to destinations throughout the body. But high insulin levels also help you store body fat—one reason that fat people often have lots of insulin in their systems. By splitting your food into six small meals a day, you can avoid the outpouring of insulin and the subsequent buildup of body fat.

What Do You Eat?

Do you eat many foods high in carbohydrates (sugar and starch)? If so, you may crave carbohydrates even though you think they're fattening or addicting. As a result, you may eat carbohydrates all the time, perhaps furtively. Do you eat a lot of fried foods? If so, you are probably accustomed to a meal that sits heavily in your stomach and lasts. You would do well to fortify your diet with extra fiber—beans, bran, fruits, and vegetables—and lots of water. These give you a sensation of fullness without contributing to health problems that can stem from excess dietary fat. Do you feel that every meal must contain a piece of sausage, bacon, or something meaty and chewy to be complete? Many meats are loaded with fat and calories, and you may want to consider experimenting with meat substitutes. Even diehard meat eaters often find that broccoli, tofu, and similar foods make delightful meat substitutes. In general, aim for variety. As a rule of thumb, try not to eat the same food twice in five days.

Where Do You Eat?

Do you find that you eat most of your meals away from the kitchen table, your dining room table, or

Variety—A Key to Healthful Eating

Variety may be more than the spice of life. It may help us regulate our appetite. Dr. Barbara Rolls, an appetite researcher at the Johns Hopkins University School of Medicine, says that a varied diet stimulates our appetites. When she gave average-weight volunteers three successive courses of pasta, the diners ate 15 percent more when each course had different-shaped pasta than when the pasta all looked the same.

How does this help someone who's trying to eat *less?* Well, boring foods could tempt you to give up on a healthful diet and slip back into old habits. If a nutritious diet is varied, it can help you stick with foods that you know are good for you.

So if you want to avoid temptation, don't confine yourself to a few healthful choices, because your plan will probably backfire. Instead, expose yourself to a full range of tasty, nutritious foods.

some other traditional dining area? Do you eat in bed? While standing? At your desk? While feeding the baby? In fast-food restaurants? Part of a strategy for healthful eating is declaring your right to sit and enjoy a meal without distractions. Pledge that you will eat whatever you choose, but that your meal must be in a dish, and you must eat it while sitting at a table.

How Do You Feel When You Eat?

Mood has a significant influence on how often we eat. Many of us eat to feed our nerves. We use food to deaden hurt, comfort fear, or calm excitement. When you keep a food diary, you may discover that you eat when you feel uncomfortable. If so, try this trick. Before you take a bite of food, take a break. Drink a glass of water or a cup of tea. Put some space—or some time—between you and the desire to soften your feelings with food. You may find that the break helps quiet your urge to eat.

Our mood also influences our hunger signals. Normal healthy people feel hunger signals when their stomachs are empty. But many of us miss these signals. We may eat constantly, never letting our stomach actually empty. Or we may dull the hunger cues with coffee or soda in an attempt to avoid eating. Or we may try to ignore the hunger by preoccupying ourselves with work. Whatever we do to try to circumvent the hunger signals can backfire. Eating nonstop keeps us from knowing when we are really satisfied. Going without food for an extended period of time can prompt us to lose control when we finally do eat. It's important to learn to recognize your hunger signals and respond to them naturally—with reasonable amounts of good, nutritious food.

MAKING FOOD CHOICES WORK

If it were easy to select the foods that are the best for us, many of us would have healthier bodies and a lot of food marketers would be out of business. But it's not, and we don't, and the food industry capitalizes on our willingness to welcome a veritable flood of tasty foods. Given this sea of temptation, how is the average person supposed to stick with a reasonable eating plan?

The goal is to make your food choices work for you. You don't have to cross off any foods from your list. Just try to expand your repertoire. That may sound defeatist. After all, the idea is to eat less, not more. But the point here is to eat with more balance. For example, if you have a passion for sweets, your sweet tooth can still keep you company. But look for other tastes to crowd out your dessert addiction. Hollow calories such as candy and soft drinks can easily be replaced with the better-quality sweets that you deserve. If you have a weakness for potato chips, recognize that they can actually fit into a plan that works for you. The trick is to set limits and really stick to them. When a 16-ounce package of chips delivers 160 calories per ounce, stick to an ounce.

To start to make food choices that work for you, track your eating for at least a week. Then examine your style of eating and set goals for what you want to change. In your overall attempt to achieve better health, you can set a primary goal to lower your calorie intake enough to lose weight. No matter how hurriedly you want to shed extra pounds, keep three simple promises to yourself: (1) eat at least 1,500 calories each day; (2) don't hope to lose more than 1 percent of your body weight each week; and (3) exercise for half an hour each day, even if it's just a brisk walk.

Once you pledge yourself to a daily pattern of modest eating and healthful exercise, bear in mind these four overall goals for food selection:

1. Choose high-fiber foods. Besides delivering great nutrition, these fill you up, thus helping you avoid using fatty foods to feel satisfied. Aim for at least 30 grams of fiber a day. (Food labels often list the amount of fiber in each serving.)
2. Choose low-fat foods. These help you avoid the one nutrient that has more calories than any other. Shoot for no more than 50 grams of fat a day. Watching your fat intake is discussed in depth below.
3. Arrange meals so that you are comfortable throughout the day. Include morning, midday, and evening meals and two snacks.

4. Have water or seltzer between meals and with each meal.

Sound simple enough? Good.

The next step is to draw up some strategies to help you meet these food-selection goals. Three such strategies—*counting grams of fat, using exchange lists*, and using a program like mine, Dr. Thompson's Weight-Control Plan—are detailed below. You can use two or three simultaneously, or you can pick and choose to find one that best suits you. You may find that one strategy suits your lifestyle more than the others, or you might decide that an all-out health assault takes all the ammunition you can muster. Decide for yourself, then go into action.

Some of these strategies call for measuring your food. This can be tedious, but bear in mind that it will help you eat less than you currently eat. There's no way to get around having to do *some* measuring and weighing, but once they get the hang of it, most people can eyeball food and get a pretty accurate sense of what it weighs. Many men and some women may feel embarrassed to weigh their food, as if doing so is humiliating or wimpish. Just remember that it's for a great cause: Your health and your life-span are at stake. Again, you can use food labels as a rough guide for the amount of food that you are handling.

If we're talking about measuring and weighing, you can probably guess that these three strategies work best for people who are relatively good with numbers and who are conscientious. It also helps if you're a person who feels comfortable with structure. If these qualities describe you, chances are the strategies will work for you.

If, on the other hand, you're more comfortable in unstructured settings, you're oriented more to the big picture than to details, or adding and subtracting just aren't your forte, you'll still benefit from keeping a food diary. Once you can see the hard facts about what you eat and when, then you can start to gradually overhaul your diet. Try different ways of preparing food—less frying and sautéing, more broiling and steaming. Try improving the quality of your foods—more vegetables and beans and whole grains, less meat and fat and refined grains. Try brown-bagging your lunch to avoid feeling captive to the office cafeteria. Try new strategies for outfoxing junk food: If a doughnut looks infinitely more desirable than an apple when the office snack cart rolls through at 3:00 every afternoon, beat it to the punch by eating your apple at 2:30.

There may be times when you would like to eat more than your plan allows. Many people find that it helps to have a strategy to guard against eating unplanned portions. You can have other foods on hand for when you get the urge for seconds. Good choices: salads, fruit, clear broth, herbal teas, sugar-free soft drinks. If you get desperate, using excessive condiments (salt, vinegar, hot sauce) will render an otherwise tempting food virtually inedible. An even better strategy: Have you ever tried giving away a portion of your food that you don't want to eat? It works.

Finally, in restaurants, remember that an ounce of prevention is worth a pound of fat. Avoid "all you can eat" buffets. They can put you in the difficult position of not only shouting down your vocal taste buds but arguing with your wallet about getting your money's worth.

On with the strategies.

Strategy 1: Count Grams of Fat

How many times have you heard people turn down a baked potato because they were on a diet? Or give up eating bread because they were watching their weight? For years, we've all assumed that starches on our lips turn to fat on our hips. Not so anymore. Now we know that starches aren't fattening at all. It's *fat* that's fattening—the sour cream that we slather onto our baked potatoes, and the butter that we spread on our bread. Fat is a necessary nutrient, but most of us overdo it. We become captivated by the sensuousness of fat, the richness it lends to desserts, the crispness that it gives fried foods. Fat also captures a good deal of the flavor in some foods. All of these reasons cause us to overuse fat, often doubling the calorie count of a meal as a result.

There Are Calories, and Then There Are Fat Calories

Let's say you have a thing for greasy foods. Sausage and eggs and hot buttered grits. Fried chicken and biscuits. Burgers and fries. They add up to, say, 3,500 calories a day. On a weeklong visit to your brother the vegetarian, your diet encounters a radical and delicious transformation—fruit salad, pinto beans and cornbread, stir-fried vegetables over brown rice. At the end of the week, you make a remarkable discovery. You've eaten just as many calories as before—3,500 a day—but you've lost weight.

That's because your body treats fat calories differently than it does carbohydrate calories. Any extra calories consumed as fat head straight for the fat cells in your belly, thighs, hips, or elsewhere. In fact, 97 percent of excess dietary fats wind up being stored in fat cells. In contrast, a lesser proportion—about 75 percent—of excess carbohydrate calories make it to the fat cells.

So you can actually lose weight by switching from a fatty diet to one high in carbohydrates—even if the calorie count in both cases is the same.

Get a handle on your fat consumption by using your food diary. Save some space in the last column to calculate the number of grams of fat and the number of calories that you consume each day. Once you have a fairly clear idea of how much fat you eat in a given day, set a goal of 50 grams or less of fat per day. Table 1 (page 145) lists the fat content of a variety of common foods. Figuring the fat level is easy for foods with a single ingredient and for packaged foods that come with labels. Mixtures, such as casseroles, are more difficult. For these, try to break down the ingredients to estimate the amount of fat.

Your daily ceiling of 50 grams of fat lets you control

How Much Fat Is on That Fork?

Fat can be clever. It's not always where we think it is. You may think you're doing well to stick with just a salad the next time you go to McDonald's. But if you douse it with four servings of McDonald's peppercorn salad dressing, you will have eaten 44 grams of fat. That's well on the way to your daily allotment of 50 grams in one fell swoop. On the other hand, many traditionally fatty products are being reformulated with little or no fat at all. Just as some salad dressings (like McDonald's) contain loads of fat, some mayonnaise (like Miracle Whip Free) and salad dressings (like Kraft Free), contain none at all. It pays to scrutinize food labels. Here are some helpful guidelines:

A. Foods with less than 1 gram of fat per serving:
   - Fruits—all
   - Vegetables—leaves, roots, flowers, pods, etc.
   - Beans and peas—all
   - Grains—rice, rice cakes, oatmeal, corn, grits, tortillas, cornmeal, flour, barley, some crackers, matzohs
   - Skimmed milk products—fat-free cheese, fat-free yogurt
   - Other (check food label)—frozen desserts made with Simplesse® or other fat substitutes, fat-free salad dressings, soft drinks, low-calorie sweeteners, gelatin desserts, angel food cake

B. Foods with 1 to 3 grams of fat per serving:
- Cereals (check labels; some granolas and other cereals have more fat)—shredded wheat, puffed cereal, flakes, bran, wheat germ
- Breads—whole wheat, white, rye, Italian, French, pita
- Lean fish*—flounder, cod, perch, whiting, porgy, tuna in water, shellfish
- Low-fat milk products—1% fat milk, low-fat yogurt
- Skinless poultry*—turkey, chicken, cornish hens
- Red meat*—hind quarter, well-trimmed beef, leg of lamb, lean pork, veal

(*as fat per ounce)

C. Foods with 4 to 6 grams of fat per serving:
- Milk products—part-skim cheeses, 2% fat milk
- Fish—mackerel, tuna in oil
- Red meat—loin cuts of beef, lamb, pork
- Spreads*—regular margarine, butter, all oils
- Desserts—cookies, low-fat ice cream
- Breads—biscuits
- Other—tofu, 1 teaspoon peanut butter

(*as fat per teaspoon)

D. Foods with 7 to 10 grams of fat per serving:
- Milk products—whole milk, hard cheese
- Desserts—cake (except for angel food), medium-fat ice cream pies
- Snacks—chips

your total intake of calories without setting you up for the "fat deprivation blues." Once our bodies are used to consuming a certain amount of fat, they signal the brain when fat consumption drops below that level. (Remember the messages sent by fat cells in Chapter 3?) If you restrict your fat consumption gradually, these urges may be less of a problem.

TABLE 1 Calorie and Fat Values for Common Foods
C = cup; T = tablespoon; oz = ounce

	Amount	Calories	Fat (g)
Milk			
Buttermilk	1 C	88	0.2
Milk, skim	1 C	88	0.2
Milk, whole	1 C	159	8.5
Vegetables			
Asparagus	4	14	0.1
Green beans, frozen, French-style	½ C	14	0.1
Beans, lima (frozen)	½ C	84	0.1
Beets	½ C	27	0.1
Beets greens, spinach, collards (cooked)	½ C	22	0.4
Brussel sprouts, frozen	½ C	30	0.4
Cabbage, raw	1 C	21	0.2
Cauliflower	½ C	15	0.1
Corn on cob, 5" (boiled)	1	70	0.8
Peas, green, frozen	½ C	55	0.3
Potato, french fried (2" to 3½" diameter)	10	137	6.6
Potato, sweet, mashed	¼ C	73	0.3
Potato, white, baked (2" diameter)	½ C	59	0.1
Pumpkin, carrots, winter squash*	½ C	37	0.3
Rutabaga, mashed	½ C	42	0.1
Summer squash	½ C	13	0.1
Celery, stalks	3	9	0.1
Cucumber, slices	16	9	0.1
Lettuce, shredded	1 C	9	0.1
Tomatoes, canned & juiced	½ C	24	0.2
Tomatoes, fresh (2⅔" diameter)	1	20	0.2
Turnips, mashed	½ C	26	0.3
Fruits			
Apple (2½" diameter)	1	61	0.6
Applesauce, unsweetened	½ C	50	0.3
Banana, medium	½	51	0.1
Berries (blue, black, raspberries)*	½ C	46	0.4
Cantaloupe (¼ of 6" diameter)	1 C	48	0.2
Orange/grapefruit juice*	½ C	54	0.1
Orange, small	1	49	0.1
Grapefruit	½	37	0.1
Cherries, large	10	47	0.2

	Amount	Calories	Fat (g)
Grapes	12	41	0.2
Pears, water pack	1	50	0.4
Raisins (1½ T)	½ oz	40	0.0
Strawberries	1 C	55	0.7
Watermelon, diced	1 C	42	0.3
Bread and Crackers, Enriched			
Biscuit (2" diameter, 1¼" high)	1	103	4.8
Cornbread, piece (2½" x 2½" x 1⅜")	1	178	5.8
Frankfurter roll (6")	1	119	2.2
Graham crackers (2" squares or 1 rectangle)	2	55	1.3
Hamburger bun (3½")	1	119	2.2
Muffin, plain (2" x 1½")	1	118	4.0
Saltines (2½" square)	4	48	1.3
Soda crackers (2½" square)	5	65	1.8
White or whole wheat bread, slice	1	76	0.9
Cereals, Enriched			
Bran flakes, 40%	½ C	53	0.3
Corn flakes	¾ C	73	0.1
Farina, cooked	½ C	51	0.1
Grits, corn	½ C	62	0.1
Oatmeal, cooked	½ C	66	1.2
Rice, cooked	⅓ C	74	0.1
Wheat, puffed	1 C	54	0.2
Pasta, Enriched			
Noodles, macaroni, spaghetti*	½ C	91	0.6
Meat, Poultry, and Fish			
Bacon, crisp, slices	2	86	7.8
Beef, lamb, veal (medium-fat)*	1 oz	79	5.2
Beef liver	1 oz	65	3.0
Bologna (1 slice, 4½" diameter)	1 oz	86	7.8
Chicken, light meat	1 oz	50	1.0
Cod, haddock, halibut (broiled)*	1 oz	48	1.8
Ham, cured (trimmed)	1 oz	61	1.0
Ham, cured (untrimmed)	1 oz	92	7.1
Hot dog	1	139	12.4
Pork, fresh (trimmed)	1 oz	72	4.0
Pork, fresh (untrimmed)	1 oz	103	8.1

	Amount	Calories	Fat (g)
Shrimp	1 oz	37	0.4
Tuna, canned in oil	1 oz	82	5.8
Tuna, canned in water	1 oz	36	0.2
Egg, large	1	82	5.8
Cheese			
Cheddar, domestic	1 oz	113	9.1
Cottage cheese, small curd, creamed	½ C	112	4.4
Cottage cheese, small curd, uncreamed	½ C	63	0.2
Peanut Butter	2 T	188	16.2
Dried Beans and Peas			
Navy beans, kidney beans, split peas*	½ C	114	0.4
Fats			
Cream, light, 20% or half & half*	1 T	26	2.5
French or Italian dressing*	1 T	75	7.6
Margarine/butter*	1 T	34	3.8
Mayonnaise, salad dressing*	1 T	83	8.8
Oils	1 T	120	13.6
Nuts			
Peanuts, pecans, walnuts, almonds*	2 T	103	9.6
Desserts			
Brownies, with nuts (1¾" x 1¾" x ⅞")	1	97	6.3
Cake, chocolate (3" x 3" x 2")	1 piece	322	15.1
Cake, plain (3" x 3" x 2")	1 piece	313	12.0
Chocolate pudding	½ C	193	6.1
Cookies, chocolate chip	2	99	4.4
Custard, baked	½ C	153	7.3
Gelatin dessert	½ C	71	0.0
Ice cream, vanilla	4 oz	129	7.0
Pie, apple (9" diameter)	⅛ pie	302	13.1
Sherbert, orange	4 oz	130	1.2
Vanilla wafers	5	93	3.2
Sweets			
Milk chocolate	1 oz	147	9.2

	Amount	Calories	Fat (g)
Molasses, jams, jelly, maple syrup*	1 T	52	0.0
Soft drinks	6 fl oz	72	0.0
Sugar	1 T	46	0.0

* Average value for the group of foods listed.

None of the foods that are fat-free (in other words, foods that contain less than 1 gram of fat) need to be measured. Only those foods that contain 1 gram of fat or more per serving need to be measured and limited by the amount of fat that you choose to enjoy at any given meal or on any given day. Fifty grams may not sound like very much, but it actually gives you a fair amount of leeway. Here, for example, is a sample menu that reveals the amount of flexibility that you can introduce in a daily budget of 50 grams of fat. Foods that do not have to be measured are marked with an asterisk (*).

	Meal	*Grams of fat*
t =teaspoon; C = cup; oz=ounce		
Morning:	Puffed rice*	0
	Skim milk*	0
	Fresh orange sections	0
	1 slice toast	1
	1 t low-fat margarine	3
	Tea or coffee (no cream) or fruit juice	0
	Water	0
Snack:	Raisins*	0
	Fat-free crackers	0
	Tea, fruit juice, or water	0
Midday:	8 oz mushroom barley soup	3
	2 slices bread	2
	2 oz turkey	6

	Meal	*Grams of fat*
t =teaspoon; C = cup; oz=ounce		
Mustard*	0	
	Large tossed salad*	0
	Fat-free dressing*	0
	Fruit juice or water	0
Snack:	Rice cakes*	0
	Vegetable juice*	0
	Water	0
Evening:	Large baked sweet potato	2
	2 t low-fat margarine	6
	4 oz skinless chicken	13
	1 C string beans	3
	Large tossed salad*	0
	1 t olive oil	5
	Vinegar*	0
	Water	0
Snack:	5 C popcorn	2
	Popped in 1 t oil	4
	Fat-free yogurt*	0
	Fat-free beverage	0
	Water	0
	Total grams of fat	**50**

Since fats are calorie-rich, watching your fat intake lets you carve from your daily diet the densest source of calories. Once you do that, you'll find it difficult to load too many calories into your day. For example, what would you do if you were asked to choose between two medium baked potatoes and one baked potato with three pats of butter? The two potatoes combined weigh in at 160 calories, whereas one potato with butter is 180. Not much difference there; skipping the buttery potato saves you only 20 calories. But if you decided to go with two potatoes, consider how full you would feel midway into the second one. You might decide after one and a half potatoes that you've had enough. That would mean you have eaten only 120 calories rather than 180 calories. A 60-calorie savings three meals a day means that in three weeks, you will have lost over one pound of weight. (Remember that one pound equals 3,500 calories; 60 calories x 3 times a day x 21 days = 3,780 calories.) Over the course of a year, you would save a surprising 65,700 calories. That's the equivalent of over 18 pounds of weight—*without being on a diet.* With a conscious effort to renovate your daily food choices, you can reach your goals quickly, and with a happy stomach.

One reason your stomach will be happier is that you are eating high-fiber foods. Fiber of all kinds gives the sense of fullness that helps you want and eat less food at each meal. Less food means fewer calories, which usually translates to weight loss. How much weight loss? Many people find that a daily regimen of 50 grams of fat turns into about 2 to 3 pounds of weight loss per month.

It's not difficult to stick to the 50-gram limit even when you dine at restaurants. If you don't have the means or the motivation to prepare your food from scratch or to measure food often, it's possible to eat healthfully away from home. When dining out, simply ask that your meal be prepared and served with no butter, cream, or fatty toppings. Many cafeterias and restaurants offer fat-free salad dressings. These make delightful toppings for baked potatoes, hot or cold vegetables, and even skinless chicken (not to mention salad). In fast-food restaurants, order fat-free muffins or standard pancakes instead of rich biscuits or croissants. If you opt for a burger, skip the cheese and "special sauce." You might get away with as few as 4 grams of fat, a pleasantly modest amount.

Conserving fat does more than protect your waistline. It protects your health. A low-fat, high-fiber diet reduces the risk of the health problems outlined in Chapter 2—heart disease, and cancer of the breast, prostate, and large intestine. It helps keep your blood pressure and your blood cholesterol low.

Low-fat foods are easy to buy, store, and prepare, and they're good for all ages. Most of all, a low-fat style of eating keeps on working for you for a lifetime.

Eating is a personal, private act that occupies a fundamental niche in our lives. Thus changing our eating habits means changing our lives. Like any change, this one takes time. We learn how to do it gradually, just as any other major life change comes in small steps. Think of how long it took you as a child to learn to walk or to read. That's the same basic life-changing process we're talking about here. It shouldn't be rushed, but it also doesn't have to be feared. Dietary changes benefit from support and encouragement. Support yourself by planning ahead. (Tips and grocery lists follow later in this chapter.) Encourage yourself with humor. Oprah used to tell her skinny friends that if they wanted to gain some weight, all they had to do was go on a diet. That way, they would add all the pounds they wanted, and more.

Strategy 2: Use Exchange Lists

Want an easy system for planning a well-balanced, moderate-calorie diet? Use exchange lists (Table 2, page 154). An exchange list is a compilation of foods, all grouped by nutritional profile. There's a vegetable family, a starch family, a milk products family, and so forth. Within each family, a portion size is given for each food item, so that any given portion delivers roughly the same amount of carbohydrates, protein, fat, and calories. That way, all you have to do is follow a simple daily plan to figure out how many food exchanges to eat. Here's a daily plan for 1,500 calories:

1,500 calories

7 starches ☐ ☐ ☐ ☐ ☐ ☐ ☐
5 proteins ☐ ☐ ☐ ☐ ☐
3 vegetables ☐ ☐ ☐
3 fruits ☐ ☐ ☐
2 milks ☐ ☐
5 fats ☐ ☐ ☐ ☐ ☐
Unlimited "free foods"

Keeping a checklist like the one above will help ensure that you stay on track as the day progresses.

You wouldn't want to eat all seven starches or three proteins in a single meal, of course. Spread them out over the entire day. Use this as a guide (t=teaspoon; C=cup; oz=ounce):

Recommended Food Exchanges		*Sample Menu*
Morning:	2 starches	½ C hot cereal 1 slice whole wheat toast

	1 fat	2 t reduced-fat (diet) margarine
	1 fruit	½ small banana
	1 milk	8 oz skim milk
	free foods	tea with sugar substitute
Midday:	2 starches	1 5" whole wheat pita
	2 proteins	2 oz tuna in water
	1 fat	2 t reduced-fat mayonnaise
	1 vegetable	¾ C vegetable soup
	free foods	large tossed salad
		fat-free dressing
		calorie-free beverage
Snack:	1 fruit	1 small apple
Evening:	2 starches	⅓ C black-eyed peas
		⅓ C rice
	3 proteins	3 oz skinless baked chicken
	2 vegetables	½ C string beans
		½ C carrots
	2 fats	2 t reduced-fat mayonnaise
		1 t olive oil
	free foods	sliced cucumbers
		calorie-free beverage
Snack:	1 starch	3 cups popcorn, popped in:
	1 fat	1 t olive oil
	1 milk	8 oz skim milk, blended with:
	1 fruit	½ banana

Turn to Chapter 8 (page 193) for more meal plans based on 1,500 calories.

Once you get the hang of it, you will find that swapping one food for another takes no effort at all. After a couple of weeks, you will be able to sort through the boxes in your head. Nevertheless, most people find it still extremely helpful to continue to record what they eat.

The beauty of exchange lists is their flexibility. When a meal calls for two starches, you can either have one cup of spaghetti, or you can "exchange" it for one-half cup mashed potatoes plus half an ear of corn. Two fruits can be either two dates and three-quarters of a cup of strawberries, or one large banana.

Likewise, if you want to allow more calories into your daily diet, you can add the equivalent in food exchanges. Let's say, for example, that you want to increase your daily intake by 300 calories. From Table 2, you can see that adding two starches, one vegetable, one fruit, and one fat gives you just about 300 calories. So you simply add these food exchanges to your checklist:

1,500 calories		+300 calories	
7 starches	☐ ☐ ☐ ☐ ☐ ☐ ☐	2	☐ ☐
5 proteins	☐ ☐ ☐ ☐ ☐		
3 vegetables	☐ ☐ ☐	1	☐
3 fruits	☐ ☐ ☐	1	☐
2 milks	☐ ☐		
5 fats	☐ ☐ ☐ ☐ ☐	1	☐
Unlimited "free foods"			

Table 2 Exchange Lists

C = Cup; T = Tablespoon; t = teaspoon; oz=ounce

List 1. Free Foods

Provides insignificant calories, protein, fat, and carbohydrates per serving.

Bouillon	Gelatin, unsweetened	Mustard	Chicory
Clear broth	Lemon, lime	Pickle, sour	Chinese cabbage
Coffee		Pickle, dill—unsweetened	Cucumbers
Tea		Vinegar	Endive
			Escarole
			Lettuce (all kinds)
			Parsley
			Radishes
			Watercress

List 2. Vegetable Exchanges = ½ C cooked (*unlimited if eaten raw)

Provides approximately 25 calories, 2 grams protein, and 5 grams carbohydrates per serving.

Asparagus
Bean sprouts
Beans (green or wax)
Broccoli*
Brussels sprouts
Cabbage (all kinds)
Carrots
Catsup (2 T)
Cauliflower
Celery
Eggplant
Mushrooms*
Okra
Onion
Peppers (red or green)*
Rutabaga
Sauerkraut
Summer squash*
Tomatoes, 1 C raw or ½ C cooked
Tomato or vegetable juice (6 oz)
All leafy greens

List 3. Fruit Exchanges

Provides approximately 60 calories and 15 grams carbohydrates per serving.

FRUITS

Apple (2")
Applesauce (½ C)
Apricots, fresh (2 medium)
Apricots, dried (4 halves)
Bananas (4½")
Blueberries (¾ C)
Cantaloupe (⅓; 5" diameter)
Cherries (12 large)
Dates (2)
Figs, dried (1½)
Fruit cocktail, canned (½ C)
Grapefruit (½ medium)
Grapes (15)
Honeydew melon (⅛; 7" diameter)
Mango (½ small)
Nectarine (1 small)
Orange (1 small)
Papaya (1 C)
Peach (1 medium)
Pear (1 small)
Pineapple (¾ C)
Prunes, dried (3, raw)
Raisins (2 T)
Strawberries (1¼ C)
Tangerine (1 large)
Watermelon, cubed (1¼ C)

JUICES

Apple, pineapple (½ C)
Grape, prune (⅓ C)
Grapefruit, orange (½ C)

List 4. Starch Exchanges

Provides approximately 80 calories, 15 grams carbohydrates, 3 grams protein, and trace fat per serving.

BREADS

Any loaf (1 slice, 1 oz)
Bagel (1 oz)
Biscuit (2½")
Tortllla (1, 6" diameter)
Waffle (1, 4½" diameter)
Bun, hamburger or hot dog (½)
Chow mein noodles (½ C)
Pretzels (¾ oz)
Rye Krisps (4)
Saltines (5)
Corn bread (1, 2" cube)
Dinner roll (1, 2" diameter)
Pastas (½ C)
Rice (⅓ C)
English muffin (½)
Muffin, plain (1 small)
Pancake (1, 4" diameter)
Stuffing (bread) (¼ C)
Potatoes, white (1 small or ½ C)
Pumpkin (¾ C)
Winter squash (1 C)

CRACKERS	CEREALS	VEGETABLES	DESSERTS
Graham, 2 (2½" square)	Hot cereal (½ C)	Beans or peas (plain) cooked, (⅓ C)	Fat-free sherbert (4 oz)
Matzoh (½, 4" x 6")	Dry flakes (¾ C)	Corn (½ C or 6" cob)	Angel cake (1½" square)
Melba toast (4)	Dry puffed (1½ C)	Parsnips (⅔ C)	
Oyster (20, ½ C)	Bran (5 T)	Plantain (½ C)	
	Wheat germ (3 T)		

List 5. Protein Exchanges (cooked weight)

Provides approximately 55 calories, 7 grams protein, and 3 grams fat per serving.

Beef, lamb, pork veal, lean only (1 oz)
Cottage cheese, uncreamed (¼ C)
Egg (1 medium)
Fish, such as whiting, cod, perch, etc. (1 oz)
Hard cheese (½ oz)
Lobster (2 oz)
Oysters, Clams, Shrimp (2 oz)
Parmesan, grated (2 T)
Peanut butter (2 t)
Poultry, without skin (1 oz)
Tuna, packed in water (¼ C)
Salmon, pink, canned (¼ C)

List 6. Milk Exchanges

Provides approximately 90 calories, 8 grams protein, trace fat, and 12 grams carbohydrates per serving.

Buttermilk, fat-free (1 C)
Skim milk (1 C)
1 % fat milk (7 oz)
Yogurt, plain, made with nonfat milk (¾ C)

List 7. Fat Exchanges

Provides approximately 45 calories and 5 grams fat per serving.

Avocado (⅛, 4" diameter)
Bacon, crisp (1 slice)
Butter, Margarine (1 t)
Chitterlings (½ oz)
French dressing (1 T)
Mayonnaise (1 t)
Roquefort dressing (2 t)
Thousand Island dressing (2 t)
Oil (1 t)
Olives (5 small)
Peanuts (10)
Walnuts (6 small)
Pecans (2 whole)
Pumpkin seeds (2 t)
Coconut, shredded (2 T)

Strategy 3: Use a Weight-Control Program

On page 114, you'll find some commonsense rules for judging whether a given dietary plan is reasonable. I've presented those rules because the purpose of this book isn't to elevate one specific dietary plan over another, but to give you the tools to make sound decisions on your own.

To show how you can take information from different weight-control programs and construct your own diet plan, I'd like to explain my own eating regimen and weight-control program, Dr. Thompson's Weight-Control Plan. You may find it—or some variation—useful or not; my only purpose is to help show how individualized a personal eating plan can be, and how it can be structured to match your personal eating style and tastes.

All good weight-control programs—and there are plenty of them—give some sort of advice on choosing food. I should know: I don't think there are three diets I haven't tried at one time or another. The actual names of the diets aren't that important; what's important is the ability to recognize valuable elements within one plan or another—those elements that seem to resonate with who you are, what your lifestyle is, and how you want to think about your health.

Before I explain the elements of my eating plan, let me place that information in context and tell you where I'm coming from. Like many people, I didn't have a weight problem as a young person. When I graduated from college, I weighed 99 pounds even though I had an excellent appetite. Eight years later when I married, my weight was 122 pounds. Then came the problems. By the time I was 43 years old, I had had five children, and although I was scrupulous about not gaining weight during the pregnancies, each birth seemed to leave me 20 pounds heavier so that after my fifth child I hit the scales at 199 pounds. That's when I started really getting serious about my weight.

In my experience as a physician who's wrestled with her own waistline, there are two key elements of a successful weight-control program.

First, you have to be ready for a complete change in attitude. If you're skeptical about any new diet that happens to come along, you're right to ask hard questions because it's true that diets by themselves don't work. But programs can. If you put your faith in a total approach to weight control, rather than focusing on food alone, you probably won't be disappointed. (That's where exercise comes in. Remember Chapter 5?)

Second, the food plan should be one that you can follow for the rest of your life. Over the years I've lost as many as 45 pounds at a time, but I wasn't prepared to make the dietary changes a permanent part of my life. So the pounds came tumbling back.

Once you can think about weight control as more than just food control, and you're committed to making permanent changes in how you live your life, you're ready for my food plan. The plan is modeled after several weight-control programs that appeal to me, including a plan recently given to me by a Caribbean doctor who specializes in the herbal treatment of disease. Be sure to check with your doctor before embarking on this or any other weight-control regimen.

Dr. Thompson's Weight-Control Plan—There is a long list of NO's for this program:

- NO beef, veal, lamb, pork, or other red meats
- NO eggs
- NO milk, cheese, ice cream, cakes, pastries, or soft drinks
- NO coffee, tea, or chocolate
- NO white sugar or honey
- NO white-flour products (bread, noodles, etc.)
- NO added fats, butter, or oils except for olive oil, noted below
- NO added salt, pepper, bouillon cubes, other seasonings
- NO sauces or gravies
- NO mayonnaise
- NO fried, barbequed, or smoked foods
- NO alcohol

This is a bare-bones eating plan. It's high in protein, fiber, vitamins, and minerals, and low in starches and fat. I like to think of the plan as the foundation of a healthful diet, one that you can carefully add to and still maintain good health and reasonable weight. More about that later.

Let me stress again that this is a plan that works for *me.* You may find that you can enjoy some of the items on this list without jeopardizing your bottom line. For example, coffee and tea don't contain a single calorie (though caffeine is a potent drug, of course, and its diuretic effect does flush beneficial water from your system). Likewise, nobody ever accused spices, in and of themselves, of making anyone fat. But I find that making it through the day without caffeinated beverages reminds me to enjoy noncaffeinated herbal teas, which are good for my overall health. (That's a good example of the holistic approach I mentioned above.) And when I avoid spicy or heavily seasoned foods, I'm often also avoiding foods that are rich in sodium and fat. Heavily seasoned foods can also enhance your appetite, which prompts you to eat more than you otherwise would.

It may seem odd for a food plan to start with a list of foods you can't eat. I admit that the list may seem pretty limiting. I find myself using my memory when I'm faced with a favorite food I know I'm not supposed to eat: Often the satisfaction of simply remembering what it's like to eat the food is enough to lead me not into temptation, and the craving passes. Remember, too, that we can train our tastebuds to adjust to new foods. Years ago when I was pregnant with my first child, my feet swelled in the last weeks of pregnancy and I was put on a salt-free diet. I wasn't sure how I would adjust to such a stringent prescription, but I got into the habit of avoiding salt. And to this day, I enjoy foods without added salt. In other words, we can train our sense of taste over time.

Here's a list of ALLOWED foods:

- Fish, chicken, turkey
- Fruit in abundance. If you have diabetes, I recommend that you drink only grapefruit juice or the apple drink described below.
- Vegetables, including greens, eggplant, and yellow squash
- Salad dishes
- Dressings made from olive oil and lemon or lime juice

- Whole-wheat bread, salt-free, occasionally
- Fresh-squeezed grapefruit juice, 2 glasses a day
- Oat and apple drink, 2 glasses a day. Recipe below. This mixture is purported to give strength. I'm not sure that it does, but I do seem to have more energy when I drink it faithfully.
- Camomile or peppermint tea.

I steam, bake, or broil, never fry. I also don't microwave, but that's more a personal preference than a nutritional concern. I live in a high-rise apartment complex in which we occasionally have the gas turned off for repairs. I did break down and buy a small microwave oven for such times, but I very rarely use it. I heat up food in my gas oven.

I also include a number of food supplements in my food plan. As with the foods, I recommend that you show this list of supplements to your doctor before proceeding with the plan. He or she may have reason to modify the dose of one supplement or another, or suggest that you not take a supplement at all. Some of these supplements help with overall body function; vitamin A for good vision, for example. Other supplements have specific weight-control benefits as listed. You can purchase these at natural-foods stores or increasingly at many drugstores and supermarkets. If you're interested, you can read up on the many benefits of these and other supplements in any of a number of affordable reference books at bookstores and libraries.

- Sulfur bitters, to aid digestion. One teaspoon in a glass of water first thing in the morning. Sulfur bitters may be difficult to find in the United

States, although it's prevalent in the West Indies. I've substituted Swedish bitters with success. They're available at health-food stores. The Swedish bitters I use contains alcohol and should not be used by persons with liver disease or a history of alcohol abuse.

The remaining supplements should be divided into two portions and taken with meals, preferably breakfast and dinner. This is a partial list of the items I was given; I've modified them for my personal use.

- Vitamin A—10,000 IU, 2 capsules a day
- Vitamin C—1,000 mg, 2 tablets a day
- B complex vitamin—2 capsules a day
- Vitamin E, 400 IU—2 capsules per day
- Garlic—270 mg, 6 tablets a day
- Gentian liquid—20 drops, 2 times a day, aids in digestion but contains alcohol
- Burdock root—540 mg, 2 capsules a day
- Yellow dock—500 mg, 2 capsules a day
- Dandelion root—475 mg, 2 capsules a day
- Brewer's yeast—7.5 grains, 2 tablets a day
- Kelp—.15 mg, 2 tablets a day, to reduce appetite. Kelp contains iodine so you shouldn't take it if you have thyroid disease.
- Hawthorne berries—510 mg, 2 capsules a day
- Goldenseal—500 mg, 2 capsules a day. A near-constant feature of herbal diets, and one that my patients have spoken of for years.
- Echinacea—300 mg, 2 capsules a day
- Calcium-magnesium supplement, 1,000 mg calcium plus 500 mg magnesium, twice a day

I also take a prescription vitamin, Berocca Plus (Roche Laboratories), 2 per day.

How I eat is as important as *what* I eat. I've picked up several ideas from various diet plans on how to go about eating:

- Count your hunger on a scale of 0 to 10. A 0 is when you're ravenous. A 10 feels like you just ate Thanksgiving dinner. The time to stop eating is when you reach the halfway mark at 5. It may take you a while to recognize this point, but as you persist, you will notice that you become uncomfortable if you eat more, and you'll come to recognize when you've had enough. The walls of the stomach are muscular, and if you reduce your food intake over time, the stomach literally shrinks. That's a good thing, because the amount of food that you could eat before you started your eating plan makes you feel uncomfortably full, and you end up eating less.
- Have at least one meal, preferably dinner, in surroundings that are comfortable and relaxed. It's good to have company if you can, so you can focus on more than just the food. I live alone, but I usually set my dinner with different pretty plates which I rotate frequently. I like to listen to music when I eat; it's relaxing and probably aids digestion. I don't talk on the phone, because that way it's too easy to eat a lot of food without being aware of it.
- Plan ahead. Check your schedule and map out how you will eat for the day. If at all possible, take your lunch to work. That way, you'll have better control over what you're eating — plus you'll save

money. I'm semiretired, and when I'm home all day, it's not difficult to plan my meals. But I work part-time three days a week, and I have a social calendar that takes me away from home for days at a time. With my weight-control plan I can eat out, and I've compiled an entire list of restaurants that I know will prepare food the way I want.

A Daily Food Plan

Upon arising, take the bitters in water.

BREAKFAST

Freshly squeezed grapefruit juice. The diet plan calls for two glasses per day but I drink only one. Usually the juice from 1½ grapefruits yields at least 8 ounces of juice. Some food-combination experts advocate not eating fruit too late in the day, because it can allegedly ferment in the stomach overnight. So I am careful not to eat fruit at night.

Oat and apple drink. Mix 2 tablespoons of rolled oats to 1 pint of water and 1 cut-up apple and put in a blender. This makes 2 glasses that are taken during the day. I modified this because I didn't want to take the apple too late in the day, and on many days I am not home to take the drink as an afternoon snack, which would be ideal So I make the drink like a cereal, which I like and find more filling. In a small blender (I use a Cuisinart) I place the apple and oats and just enough water to give the consistency of cereal. If you like sweets the way I do, you'll discover that certain varieties of apples are sweeter than others and that the taste of the cereal can vary accordingly.

Herbal drink. The grapefruit juice and oat drink are my breakfast. Then I take half of my supplements with camomile or peppermint tea. If I have time, I like to give myself about 45 minutes to an hour between the juice and the drink, on the advice of food-combination specialists who avoid mixing the two. On mornings when my schedule doesn't permit such a relaxed pace, I take the two simultaneously.

LUNCH

A large green salad
Allowed vegetables
Chicken, fish, or turkey
Peppermint tea (I avoid camomile during the day because it makes me sleepy)

Lots of people wonder how they can stick to their eating plan if they happen to go out to eat. Here's a menu that you can eat in virtually any restaurant. I order a house salad without dressing, and if the server can't bring oil and lemon or lime juice, I ask for a little oil and vinegar. I keep a few teabags in my purse in case the restaurant doesn't carry herbal blends. Baked chicken is on may restaurant menus; I order it without gravy and stuffing, and I remove the skin. Steamed or grilled fish is also readily available. I find that most portions are so large that I take home a doggy bag for an easy lunch or dinner for another day. Notice that the amounts to eat are not specified in this plan, but remember the rule and try not to overeat.

DINNER

Soup. The only soups I eat are the ones I make; it's difficult to know what goes into restaurant soups. Here's one of my favorite recipes:

Chicken Vegetable Soup

This is a simple, easy, flavorful soup that calls for essentially just four ingredients:

One package of soup-stock vegetables, which I get from the produce section of my supermarket.

Carcass of a baked chicken. Whenever I bake a chicken, I place the carcass in the freezer so it is ready to make soup.

Vegetables. Use what appeals to you. I use celery, shredded cabbage, chopped okra, turnips, broccoli tips, mushrooms, string beans, or Italian beans.

Herbs from Provence. This sounds fancy, but all I'm talking about here are dried thyme, rosemary, sage, and basil. This wonderful herb blend comes from Provence, France, and if you're lucky enough like me to have a friend who travels there or if you visit yourself, you can get large packages for very reasonable prices. Otherwise, just mix up your own. I also sprinkle my chicken with the herbs before baking.

Place all ingredients in a large soup pot, cover with water, and simmer until the vegetables are tender. I like to freeze this soup in smaller portions for later use.

A Large Green Salad
Chicken, fish, or turkey
Vegetables, at least three to four steamed or baked. Most of my vegetables are fresh, but I also use frozen vegetables if my careful reading of the label shows no added salt or other ingredients.
Peppermint or camomile tea

In addition to these three meals, I drink 6 to 8 glasses of spring water throughout the day.

RESULTS

I've noted a tremendous improvement in my physical and emotional well-being since I started my program. I'm more energetic: I don't wake in the morning reluctant to get out of bed and wondering how soon I'll return there. My digestion is also much improved. I used to be plagued by terrible diarrhea that stopped as soon as I went on my food plan. The culprit, I realized, was cheese. After being on the program for a month I "treated" myself to a good-sized cheese sandwich, and the diarrhea returned. And so I've put cheese on my memory list.

When you've reached your desired weight on this plan, you stick with the food program and cautiously add foods you haven't been eating. You also continue with your exercise regimen. While going through weight reduction, I weighed myself once a week, usually on Monday morning. I still do this. Then I adjust my eating for the coming week depending on whether my weight has increased, decreased, or stayed the same. If I have gained, I return to the original plan until I drop the extra pounds. If I have lost weight that week—which sometimes happens because of a busy schedule—I then make an effort to add more food in the coming week. If my weight is stable I stay the course.

When I obtained my desired weight, I evaluated what I missed most. The first thing I added was whole wheat bread. Then I added reasonable amounts of pasta or rice and an occasional baked potato, all the while adhering to the feeling of fullness. When I travel, I take my small Cuisinart with me to make the apple drink. I also found a small stainless steel juicer with a small bowl attached, so I can enjoy my grapefruit juice wherever I am.

WEIGHT MAINTENANCE

If you have set a target weight and achieved it, the challenge now facing you is keeping your weight where you want it. For some, the excitement is in the chase. As the pounds slip away, they watch the mirror to find their body's contours changing every week, and they feel their clothing becoming increasingly roomy. Those in themselves are powerful motivators that invariably help people stay focused on attaining their weight goals.

But what happens next is key. You may have proudly reached your goal, shedding 5 or 50 pounds successfully. And you may be ready to return your food scale to its home next to the fondue set that you never use. But think for a moment: How will you maintain the changes in eating and lifestyle that you now call your own? The answer is *balance*.

The strategies outlined in this chapter are designed to bring balance to your eating. If your relationship with food has been unhealthy, you may have learned to use food as a substitute for comfort, love, or support. You may have gotten into the habit of using food for recreation or for excitement. If you needed calm, you ate. If you needed rest, you ate. If you needed food, you ate. You ate in response to so many different factors that you lost track of what it means to eat when you're hungry. That's not balance.

Balance means stability and harmony. It means responding appropriately to any given emotional or physical state. It means resting when you're tired, relaxing when you're stressed out, exercising when you feel energetic. In these last two chapters, you have learned how to incorporate exercise and good nutrition in a sensible plan for better health. With a little persistence, you will find that this plan helps you shed some extra pounds as well. To stay at your desired weight, you deserve to stay in balance.

You may have heard people claim that it costs more to eat well. But a low-fat, high-fiber diet is very economical. Once you commit yourself to low-fat sources of protein, you may find yourself bypassing meats—some of the most expensive items in the supermarket. The money you save on meat can be used to buy produce. Fruits and vegetables should be dietary staples, not luxuries. Beans, peas, rice, and pasta are very affordable. You may find that adhering to your new eating plan means that you double your purchases of these foods. Still, if your food bill doesn't shrink, it should at the very worst remain the same.

What should shrink is your body weight. And what

should increase is the number of times you will say to admiring friends, "...Yes, I *have* lost an inch or two. How? I just made a few changes in how I eat. And I walk half an hour every day. Yes, I'm pleased about it myself."

CHAPTER 7

Helping Our Kids Fight Fat

It's a muggy summer afternoon in Washington, D.C., and a group of black friends have met for a softball game on the Mall, one of the few grassy areas downtown. Both teams are playing hard, and passersby stop to enjoy the game. Suddenly a coach looks up and calls a break in the action. A young black teenager is inadvertently strolling across left field. She is fat. Everyone stops to watch her. "Get along there, heavy," the coach calls out affectionately. Realizing she is the center of attention, the girl is momentarily embarrassed. But she holds her head high and shuffles from center stage, safely out of the way of errant line drives.

It's just a small moment that comes and goes. But it's heavy with symbolism. It touches on questions of self-esteem and acceptance of overweight children by the African-American community, and by society at large. Here in the shadow of the White House, where President Kennedy and his sports-minded family brought millions of youngsters new enthusiasm for physical fitness, the incident drives home how many of today's children would rather spectate than participate. And it's a reminder that while some of today's African-American adults are becoming concerned about our weight, the good health of our children—tomorrow's adults—presents a different set of challenges.

And those challenges are numerous. Black children face many of the same stresses that their parents face, but they have less power to resolve them. Violence, drugs, school failure, homelessness, physical and sexual and emotional abuse—every modern social problem bears heavily on the black child. Poor children are disproportionately African-American; only 15 percent of all children under six are black, but a full one-third of all poor children are black. For these children, extra social stresses are compounded by inadequate health care—uncoordinated social services, lackluster health promotion, not enough doctors and hospitals.

Despite the stresses—challenges that might tempt anyone to overeat or veg out as a coping mechanism—black boys on average are no heavier than their white counterparts. Around 10 percent of black males age six to seventeen are overweight, according to a 1998 study by the Centers for Disease Control. That's about the same proportion as white boys. Now, black girls are a different situation altogether. Somewhere around 16 percent of our girls are overweight. That's twice the obesity rate seen in the white girls.

As in adults, obesity presents children with a host of difficult problems, both emotional and physical. Part of the emotional burden of being overweight stems from the stigma that we associate with it. Studies show that when given a choice, children as young as kindergarteners prefer to play with kids in wheelchairs or who have serious physical handicaps rather than with fat children. Chubby children learn from a very early age that they are different—a message that can be frustrating and alienating. "People who have a different body size always stand out," Pat Swift told the *Boston Globe.* Swift is founder of the New York–based Plus Models Management Ltd., which supplies the fashion industry with models who wear sizes 14 to 24. "I just wanted to be like everyone else. I knew my *body* was different. But I, the person, wasn't different."

That self-acceptance may be a message that black children learn more easily than whites. African-American youngsters seem much less inhibited and ashamed about their weight than white children are. And studies suggest that being fat does little injury to a black child's self-esteem. When nearly 1,000 inner-city black youngsters in Philadelphia took self-esteem tests, overweight children scored a bit lower than slender ones, but all scores fell within the normal range. That may be because their parents and other black adults, who are more likely than whites to be hefty themselves, are more accepting of obesity and subscribe to a cultural standard that differs from the white ideal.

The physical risks are a different story. The physical risks of obesity in general are just beginning to draw attention from researchers; Dr. William Dietz of Boston's New England Medical Center says that's because for years researchers have avoided fat people just like the general public does. But the few specialists in the growing field of pediatric obesity tell us that fat children are prone to develop many of the same health disorders that plague fat adults: heart disease, hypertension, Type 2 diabetes, and to a lesser extent, orthopedic problems and lung infections.

It's rare to see children die from these health disorders. But the trouble is, overweight children are likely to grow up to be overweight adults. And the longer children are fat, the greater their chances of being fat when they're fully grown. Forty percent of chubby seven-year-olds will be overweight adults, as will 70 percent of chubby preadolescents. That's sobering news indeed, because adults who were fat as kids suffer from more diseases at an earlier age than do people who were average-weight children, and they die sooner.

Now that the risks of children carrying too much body weight are coming into focus, investigators are digging to uncover the reasons for this recent deluge of excess weight. And what they're finding is a slew of factors that, taken together, seem to explain why our children are growing in two directions—out as well as up.

Some of the evidence points to a genetic link. Children with unusually slow metabolisms—a condition that might be passed from parents to child—tend to gain weight. And there's more. One doctor who examined the medical records of thousands of adopted children found an interesting trend: Adopted kids were about as fat or as thin as their biological parents. Environmental factors—where the children live, how they eat, how much exercise they get—didn't seem to matter very much. In fact, "It was as if all environmental factors washed out," University of Pennsylvania psychiatrist Dr. Albert Strunkard told the *New York Times*. Dr. Strunkard suggests that perhaps one-third of our children are genetically prone to obesity.

If that's true, then kids who have a biological tendency for obesity are in the minority. Most children are fat because of their surroundings, not their genes. How can surroundings influence a kid's weight? Let's count the ways.

Reason 1: Too Much Television

Guess how much television the average two-year-old child watches each week. Two hours? Three?

Would you believe twenty-five hours? It's true. Some children watch more than that. Before television, kids spent much of their free time playing, running, exploring, bike riding. There were dozens of ways to burn calories. Nowadays, the primary interest in many children's lives is dozens of cable television stations. Between dance shows on BET, music videos on MTV, and soap operas on ABC, CBS, and NBC, today's kids have a limitless supply of entertainment, all of it free for the asking to anyone who can find a sofa to park on. Unfortunately, too few parents intervene. "The problem is not just that the child is obese," said adolescent psychiatrist Dr. Derek Miller in a *Chicago Tribune* interview, "but that he is a couch potato and as a couch potato, he is isolated and doing nothing, and the parents don't care."

Inactivity is just half the problem. What kids watch induces them to eat—and we're not talking tofu and carrot sticks here. Chocolate-dipped candy bars, sugary breakfast cereals, greasy pizza — it's a nutritionist's nightmare. "Television viewing promotes inactivity and food consumption," says Dr. William Dietz, an associate professor of pediatrics at Tufts University. And food ads, about half of which are directed at children, are partly to blame. In fact, in a move spearheaded by Dietz, the American Academy of Pediatrics has gone so far as to call for the *elimination* of all food ads aimed at kids. Dietz says American children are greatly influenced by what he terms "a tightly woven net of commercialism."

If you're wondering what the good doctor is referring to, let your mind travel back a few years to the Teenage Mutant Ninja Turtles phenomenon. At the height of the craze, there were *2,000* licensed Teenage Mutant Ninja Turtles products competing for children's attention. Some of them were innocent enough—Teenage Mutant Ninja Turtles lunch boxes, for example. But once your child had that lunch box, it was only natural to fork over a few dollars for Teenage Mutant Ninja Turtle breakfast cereal (which was 33 percent sugar). Who knows how many middle-aged African-Americans in the year 2040 will owe their tooth decay, heart disease, obesity, and other health problems to being captivated by the Teenage Mutant Ninja Turtle craze as kids?

If you doubt that commercials influence children, listen to how a bright four-year-old child named Emily explained television to *Chicago Tribune* columnist Joan Beck: "There are programs for grownups, and there are programs for children," Emily said. "The ones for children are called commercials."

Reason 2: Too Little Physical Activity

Television watching is only the first ingredient in the fattening of the American child. Physical education—or lack of it—is a close second. Not too long ago, children of all colors were caught up in a national zeal for fitness. Prompted partly by the President's Council on Physical Fitness and Sports, schoolchildren across the country were proudly huffing and puffing their way through sit-ups, pull-ups, and laps around the track. Today, fully 40 percent of all boys age six through twelve—and 70 percent of all girls age six through seventeen—can't do a single pull-up! The Chrysler Fund and the Amateur Athletic Union periodically team up to administer a four-part fitness test to a sampling of American teenagers and younger children. In 1980, 43 percent of the children managed to complete the test. In 1989, just nine years later, barely 32 percent were able to finish it.

We can thank our schools' declining emphasis on physical education for part of this disappointing news. Phys ed just isn't being taught like it used to be. No federal law compels states to offer physical education classes, and just one state — Illinois — requires all schoolchildren from first graders to high school seniors to take physical education every day. Two-thirds of fifth through twelfth graders don't have daily physical education classes, according to the American Academy of Pediatrics. And most younger children take phys ed just once or twice a week. Children who never learn the basics of exercise and sports may grow up feeling alienated from their bodies. And if they happen to be overweight, this lack of basic information about how the body works may make them reluctant to start an exercise program.

Reason 3: Family Stresses

Every family faces stresses. Some are trivial (a child losing his report card), others traumatic (a breadwinner losing his job). In most families, the fun times balance the hard times. But some children grow up barraged by chaos. Adults are unreliable, meals are unpredictable, children are unsupervised, abuse or other family violence is unremitting.

Such unstructured family environments are fertile ground for adolescent obesity, according to Dr. Laurel Mellin, an assistant professor of pediatrics and family and community medicine at the University of California at San Francisco. When Mellin examined twenty-four obese teenagers, she discovered that 46 percent—nearly half—had chaotic family lives. In the general population, only 14 percent of adolescents live in such difficult family environments. When children are surrounded by confusion and disorder, their need for comfort and security may point them toward food.

It can happen to poor families or rich, white or black. Families as a whole have become increasingly fluid in recent years, Mellin points out. "There are many more single-parent households, two-career families, and families with much less input from the extended family." When living situations become too stressful, a structured, secure family setting may be difficult to create and sustain. And a health-oriented lifestyle becomes outright impossible. "You can think about what it takes to support a child to develop healthy exercise and eating habits," Mellin told a meeting of the North American Association for the Study of Obesity. "It's much easier to go for the pizza and television than the balanced meals and tennis lessons."

Reason 4: Inappropriate Use of Food by Parents

Have you ever heard a parent coax an unruly child by saying, "I'll buy you an ice cream cone if you behave"? It may sound like a harmless act by a desperate parent. But it might unwittingly sow the seeds of a weight problem. Rewarding a child with sweets sends a parental message that ice cream, cookies, and candy bars are better than other foods. We need to help children develop a sense of balance here. A child's natural sweet tooth will drive him or her to sugary treats as it is; we don't need to give our children even more sanction to help keep the sugar industry in business.

Moreover, children need to develop the healthy habit of eating when they're hungry. When you reward children with food, they end up eating when they score well on a test, when they clean up their room, or when they're civil to their siblings, in addition to eating at mealtimes and snack times. Their food cues can get confused, and the next thing you know they've lost track of when it's appropriate to eat.

Instead of rewarding children with food, it makes more sense to reward them with praise. Or a special privilege, like getting to stay up past their normal bedtime.

It's not always easy to use food appropriately. The stress of poverty can lead parents to teach children bad eating habits. "Many parents use food as a pacifier, and many poor parents use it for a sense of well-being," Dr. Therman Evans told *Ebony*. "That is, if they have a lot of food on the table at every meal, then everything must be okay. The parents will overeat and they will urge the children to do the same." When youngsters eat too much, their fat cells swell to hold the extra calories, and their bodies produce new fat cells, thereby setting the stage for even more weight gain. Once the body makes extra fat cells, those cells can expand or shrink as the child's calorie intake dictates, but the fat cells never go away.

Growing up poor can teach kids to eat opportunistically, too. "I still remember the hard times," recalled Maryetta Wesley, an Oklahoma City mother of five, in an *Ebony* interview. "We didn't know anything about eating 'right'; all we were interested in was not being hungry. We'd eat as if there wouldn't be anything for the next day. And sometimes we were right. My mother would make us eat everything we put on our plates, and even now, forty or so years later, I still have this feeling that I have to eat everything in sight because I might not have a meal tomorrow." At the time of the interview, Wesley was "something like sixty pounds overweight." It all goes to show how childhood patterns, for better or worse, can grow to become lifelong eating habits. And that what's appropriate in one setting can turn out to be bad news in another.

Those of us who've learned a cultural tolerance for obesity should take care not to overfeed our children. Even in infancy, feeding patterns can make their mark on a child later in life. That's according to Dr. Douglas Lewis, who discovered that newborn monkeys fed 30 percent more infant formula than normal grew up to have four times as much body fat as other monkeys by the time the animals reached adolescence. Lewis, a researcher at San Antonio's Southwest Foundation for Biomedical Research, says that adolescent girls who put on weight after puberty may have been overfed as infants. (Overfeeding may not have as much of an effect on boys, because during adolescence their bodies produce more muscle and less fat.) The first two years of life seem to be the critical period for the development of fat cells. Once children are overfed during these crucial years there can be problems later on. The bottom line is to be careful about feeding an infant too much. "When the baby turns the bottle away, he may be saying that he has had enough," Dr. Lewis told a meeting of the American Heart Association.

AN OUNCE OF PREVENTION

Health professionals, alarmed by the fattening of our youth, are beginning to take childhood weight problems very seriously. Throughout the country, physicians and others are speaking out to encourage all children, no matter what they weigh, to have a healthy, long life by developing a sound relationship with food and a habit of regular, vigorous exercise.

The best way to handle childhood weight problems is to prevent them from happening. How does one go about doing that? Here's what the experts recommend:

Respect a child's food needs. This starts the day a child is born. Infants are born with a well-tuned sense for food. When they're hungry, they let you know by crying. They turn to a nipple with an open mouth and suck until they've had enough. Once they're full, they'll spit the nipple out. If you offer more milk, the child won't show any interest. Infants have a natural, inborn sense of when they need food and when they don't. Parents disturb this instinctive sense when they insist on putting a nipple to a child's mouth after the infant is finished feeding. Or when they remove the nipple before the child is through. Either way creates anxiety in a child, and turns a pleasurable, natural act into something more alarming. In time, a young child can learn to associate food with anxiety. Who's to say that a child confronted later in life by anxious circumstances—moving to a new neighborhood, studying for a difficult test—might not revert to eating, even when they're not hungry? Respect a child's food signals. It will help the child keep intact the healthy, self-regulating food sense they were born with.

Make family mealtimes sacred. Sharing meals as a family is important. Children whose families share regular mealtimes look forward to these times in the day when they can ask questions, be heard, and receive nurturing and support. If children can't get this nurturing from within the family, they'll look elsewhere. Some find it inside a refrigerator.

Mealtimes should be an enjoyable break from stressful activities of the day. If children are reading when they sit down to eat, ask them to put their books aside. If a radio or television is on, turn it off. If you feel tension or an argument brewing, resolve it before or after the meal. Tension at the table causes upset stomachs and interferes with digestion. But more important, it spoils a sacred time, a time for family members to be together as a family, to learn about each other, to teach one another, to enjoy each other.

Teach children to be aware of their food. Teach a child to chew food thoroughly and to eat slowly. Children who become aware early on of the taste and texture of food may be less apt in later years to simply eat without regard for what they're putting in their mouths. Encourage a child to develop this awareness by trying to identify a food with their eyes closed. If your young child insists on wolfing down meals, announce a contest to see how small a piece they can cut their food into. It will slow them down and help them feel full before they overeat.

Let children have occasional treats. Keeping an eye on a child's diet is an excellent idea, but well-intentioned parents can go too far. If you're iron-fisted about it, rules can backfire. Children become curious about forbidden foods. Laying down the law on ice cream sometimes creates such a fixation that all a child can think about is hot fudge sundaes. Instead of outlawing treats entirely, let a child have them in moderation. Control the portion size and how often it's served. Let a child have a small sundae once or twice a week instead of a large one every other night. And be creative about modifying treats to make them more wholesome. Buy low-fat frozen yogurt instead of ice cream for those sundaes, and use fresh-fruit toppings like bananas, berries, and sliced peaches instead of sugary syrups.

Encourage natural exercise. Children are born with very little awareness of their bodies. They know when they're in pain, when they're hungry, and when they're tired, but that's about it. Our job as parents is to help children cultivate an awareness of their bodies so they can be friends with their physical selves. That's especially important for those of us who live in cities or in neighborhoods whose yards are too small to accommodate a child's natural love of running and climbing. As children grow older, their need to explore the world becomes increasingly strong. We thwart this need when we allow our kids to park in front of a television with a bowl of snacks. There are lots of ways to instill in a child a love of physical activity:

- If you have a yard, make it kid-friendly. Think of your most pleasant outdoor childhood memories. Chances are your child will enjoy the same things, whether it's swinging from a tree branch, climbing a knotted rope, or tossing a child-sized basketball into a hoop.
- If you live in a city or your yard isn't large enough

for children, make frequent trips to nearby parks and other recreational facilities, such as YMCAs and YWCAs, lakes, and campgrounds. It gives kids a chance to run free and release energy that would otherwise stay bottled up. Even sidewalks can become centers of joyous physical activity; playing hopscotch and swinging jump ropes can entertain children for hours.

- Encourage sports, but emphasize the value of the child, not the importance of winning. Sports can be a tremendous builder of stamina, muscle strength, hand-eye coordination, and concentration—all of which can benefit a child in other parts of life. But sports can also be disruptively competitive. The teasing and taunting of children who are slower or smaller or fatter than others can hurt their self-esteem and encourage them to withdraw from sports, thus contributing to inactivity and weight problems. Keep sports fun; Lord knows children will have enough competition to deal with once they grow up.
- Exercise with your child. Every child likes to do things with a parent. If being with a parent is fun, then what the child does with the parent can be fun. And that can set the stage for years of willing exercise even after a child has grown up. (Besides, kids need guidance. Children who are especially anxious to make school sports teams have been known to sit on radiators in an effort to lose weight.)

"Every child over five will benefit from some kind of formal exercise routine," suggests David Carroll, author of *Spiritual Parenting* (Paragon House, 1990). Carroll writes of a father who takes ten minutes every morning to stretch with his child. Together they touch their toes, lift their arms to the sky, twist their heads and shoulders from side to side, do jumping jacks and push-ups and sit-ups. Sometimes they finish by running in place for a few moments or jogging around the room. It's a special time for parent and child to share the joy of movement and the specialness of each other's company.

To reap the many benefits of exercise, children, like adults, should aim for a goal of twenty to thirty minutes of continuous vigorous exercise at least three times a week. If a child is just starting off, let her body become accustomed to the extra activity gradually. Start the child with gentle stretching and five or ten minutes of walking before (warm-up) and afterward (cool-down) to allow the body an easy transition. In between, any number of calisthenics and aerobic exercises will do the trick. Examples: running in place, toe touches, jumping rope, pushing against a wall, clenching and relaxing the eyes and fists.

- Encourage dancing. Kids of all ages love to dance. Even at an early age, a child will dance spontaneously to music if given the chance. In fact, some parents discover that turning on a record is a great way to break a child out of a foul mood. Writer David Carroll says that with a little imagination, dancing can excite a child's imagination as it works his muscles. "Play fast carnival music and have children pretend they are circus performers. Play music of different moods — slow, fast, happy, scary, brave, delerious — and have children make up a dance story for each," Carroll suggests. Let children imagine that they're in Africa, and get them to enact different animal personalities: a lion, an elephant, a chicken, a giraffe. Or change the music quickly from rap to a march to a waltz to jazz to symphony, and have children make up appropriate dances for each.

One last thing: Let young children fidget. For one thing, it burns calories—up to 800 calories a day, according to investigators at the National Institutes of Health. Unless it's simply too distracting (like in church), a child's constant motion is a good thing. It doesn't mean he's nervous and it doesn't neccessarily signal a discipline problem. Children simply have to drum their fingers and tap their toes and move their arms and legs and bodies. Some believe that a child's constant motion comes from an energy deep within them, the same energy that propels them upward in stature and breadth as they grow. Instead of stifling that good energy, find a way to channel it. Exercise is a logical outlet. Encourage older children to take up chores that involve body movement: vacuuming, sweeping, raking leaves, washing a car.

HELPING CHILDREN LOSE WEIGHT

Just as there are lots of reasons that kids gain weight, there are also lots of ways to help them lose it. If you suspect that a child is eating too much because of a problem in his or her life, try to find out what the problem is and address it. Is the child distressed because his best friend is moving away? Is she being bullied in school? Abused at home? Is he worried about not being very popular with his classmates? Like adults, children can turn these stresses inward and take them out on their bodies, particularly if they have learned (as abused children typically do) to separate themselves from their bodies. It's the only way they can remove themselves from a situation too painful to remain fully present for.

If a child's weight isn't stress-related, it may stem from the child's lifestyle. As we've seen, poor eating and exercise habits can add layers to a child's middle faster than you can say "Big Mac." The researchers who are investigating childhood weight loss are overwhelmingly white; sad to say, their research has focused largely on white children. Nevertheless, let's assume that children of all colors can benefit from similar advice. Here are a few tips:

Modify the child's television habits. Limit a child's television watching to two hours a day or less, preferably during a time of the day after the child has already been active. Whether to allow exceptions to this rule is up to you; some families permit extra viewing providing children do calisthenics or other exercises as they watch. Establish a rule that there will be no snacking while watching. That way, kids won't be able to plow through food without thinking about it. Help children reduce the role of television in their lives by encouraging other activities to replace it: games, reading, quiet conversation, going for a walk, practicing a sport.

When children do watch television, make it a point to join them when you can. Point out misleading messages, such as children whom commercials portray as remaining miraculously slender despite fistfuls of pizza and no exercise.

Resist diets. This advice won't surprise you if you've read Chapter 4. Diets are notoriously self-defeating. Not only do they fail to bring permanent weight loss, but they usually cause weight gain. With children, diets pose additional problems. When parents exert too much control over their children's eating habits, kids can lose track of their own food cues, their internal sense of being either hungry or satisfied. Without these cues, children have a difficult time regulating their food intake for themselves—the ultimate goal of a good weight-control regimen. A better strategy is to enlist a child's cooperation and work together to structure a sensible program of eating and exercising that works for the child.

Overly severe food restrictions can also cause a child physical harm. Remember, childhood is a time for growth. By the age of two, children achieve half of their adult height, according to the National Center for Health Statistics. They have an extraordinary need for nutrients, and without them, a child's development can suffer. In 1987, researchers at Long Island's North Shore University Hospital were asked to investigate eight toddlers who had failed to grow normally. Well-intentioned parents had restricted the children's calories, fearing they would get fat.

Children themselves sometimes develop an unhealthy fear of obesity. When researchers at North Shore University Hospital evaluated two hundred children who were too short for their age or who had failed to begin puberty, they found that fourteen of the children were so determined to be thin that they had accidentally malnourished themselves. The children habitually skipped meals, and they ate only two-thirds of a normal daily calorie intake. Doctors worry that children who go to such lengths to deny themselves food may run the risk of developing anorexia nervosa. Clearly, it's far better to develop a positive attitude about food, eating good food in moderation, than to view it as the enemy.

Involve the family in weight loss. Being fat is a family affair. Losing fat should be, too.

If a child is overweight, chances are that one or both parents are overweight, too. There's also a pretty good chance that the entire family is sedentary, eats foods that aren't particularly good for them, and eats a lot. Children don't have control over the food that a parent buys for the family and how it is prepared, so placing on the child the burden of eating a healthful diet is asking a bit much. And asking children to both eat well and exercise more, when they watch their parents mow through a bucket of fried chicken and then park themselves on the couch, is guaranteed to fail or even to build resentment in a child.

As a parent, remember that a child's good habits start with you. Leonard Epstein and Sally Squires, authors of *The Stoplight Diet for Children*, tell a story about a family whose favorite seafood restaurant served french fries with every entree. The mother recalls that when her son realized what sticking to his eating plan would entail, he was taken aback. "The first time we went there, John was really disappointed about not being allowed to eat the french fries. But he noticed that I ordered a baked potato. The next time we went, I reminded him that he could have a baked potato instead of the french fries and he was really pleased."

In Philadelphia, black mothers and daughters showed the importance of family involvement when they enrolled in a University of Pennsylvania program called WRAP (Weight Reduction and Pride). The girls, all twelve to sixteen years old and from poor or lower-middle-class backgrounds, had an average weight of 209 pounds. Over the course of four months, the daughters and many mothers attended weekly sessions that taught them how to measure and record their food intake, make wise food choices, and assemble well-balanced meals of 1,000 to 1,500 calories per day. The participants picked up tips on limiting the number of places where they ate, and on eating slowly. They also learned to change self-defeating attitudes about their weight and to step up their level of physical activity. The emphasis was on modifying the children's lifestyle, not dieting.

At the end of the four-month period, children who had attended the sessions by themselves lost an average of 4 pounds. But girls whose mothers had attended the same sessions but at different times than their daughters lost 7 pounds. And daughters who attended sessions with their mothers lost 8 pounds. All of the children became healthier, both physically and emotionally. The combination of eating well and getting more exercise trimmed their body fat, dropped their blood pressure, and reduced their cholesterol levels. And all children ended the study with less depression and more self-esteem. But the girls who lost the most weight were those whose mothers were involved in the process alongside them.

What happens when parents try to lose weight along with their children? The children lose more weight. That's according to research at the University of Pittsburgh, where chubby children and their overweight parents attended regular weekly meetings on diet and exercise. The parent-child partnerships were divided into three groups. The first group was promised a reward (a cash rebate for the parent; a trip to the zoo and other special activities for the child) for simply attending the instruction sessions. The second group was rewarded if the child lost weight. The third group was rewarded if both parent and child lost weight.

In the end, the kids whose parents were eating good food and pulling on sweatpants right beside the children lost a significant amount of weight. The children in the other two groups actually *gained* weight. How's that for the power of family togetherness?

If you need more help, look into an organized weight-control program. Obviously, a dedicated, supportive family effort can do a lot to help a child reduce his or her weight. And the better eating habits, combined with a vigorous program of exercise, will benefit the entire family, not just the child. If you find that a child is still struggling to lose weight, even after consulting with a doctor and trying an unsupervised weight-control effort at home, think about enrolling in a formal program. There are lots of programs around, and although they can be expensive, they may be able to provide just the guidance and group support that your child (and you) need. Look for a program that involves parents and doesn't promise quick weight loss. There should also be some involvement by a physician or a hospital. Try local hospitals or medical schools; sometimes these offer weight-loss programs as part of their health promotion efforts.

Most of all, give a child love. Work with your child. Praise him when he tries hard. Be supportive when she slips. Encourage her to keep at it.

Like many black adults, black children often grow

up feeling that they have little voice over their destiny and that their lives are largely beyond their control. The countless stresses that rain down upon our children make that assumption easy to understand. But if there's one fact that emerges from programs designed to teach black kids about health, it's that our children are eager to learn. That message has come through loud and clear in a project called "Know Your Body." The brainchild of the New York–based American Health Foundation, "Know Your Body" introduced thousands of black schoolchildren across the country to basic information about disease prevention and health promotion. Kids learned about the importance of exercise and a good diet. They learned the dangers of smoking. They learned how to prevent heart disease, cancer, and hypertension — the three biggest killers of African-Americans and of all Americans.

And once the children understood, they acted. In New York City, black children enrolled in the "Know Your Body" program lost weight, had lower cholesterol levels, and experimented less with cigarette smoking. In Washington, D.C., black children lowered their blood pressure and cholesterol levels, and increased their physical fitness. "We found that black children are just as interested in their health as white or Hispanic children are," says Dr. Ken Resnicow, chief of child health research for the American Health Foundation. "In fact, black adolescents who stay in school have better health profiles than white adolescents do. They smoke less and they use fewer drugs."

Our children have shown us that when they're armed with accurate information and a sense of hope, they're willing to take charge of their health for the better. Our job is to provide the encouragement and support that can make it all happen.

CHAPTER 8

Menus for Healthful Weight Loss

GENERAL RECOMMENDATIONS FOR USING THE MENUS

The menus total approximately 1,500 to 1,600 calories each day. Include a dessert or snack that has about 100 calories. Good ideas for low-calorie desserts/snacks include sugar-free gelatin, 1 generous cup (C) of fresh fruit salad, one large baked apple (see recipe on Day 2), 1 cup sorbet, ¾-inch slice of angel food cake, or three fig bars. See package labels for additional ideas.

Have a salad at every evening meal. It should be made up of a variety of lettuces (such as Boston, Romaine, iceberg, etc.), and at least three other raw vegetables (such as radishes, red or green bell pepper, carrots, scallions, cucumber, etc.). The amount of salad is unlimited. Use approximately 2 tablespoons (T) of reduced-fat salad dressing.

Use reduced-fat margarine and mayonnaise at the table and in preparation. If you prefer full-fat margarine, mayonnaise, or butter, simply use half as much as the menu calls for.

If you use skim milk instead of 1% fat milk, include an additional ½ teaspoon (t) of regular margarine or oil *or* 1 teaspoon of reduced fat margarine.

The menus reflect typically available and popular foods and offer simplified or slightly embellished old favorites. Substitute the closest version of a sandwich filling or main dish when necessary. Always eat at least the amount of food that is recommended; very low calorie plans make losing more difficult. Be flexible and move any food from a meal to make it a snack.

Where rice is suggested, try brown rice as often as possible.

DAY 1 ■ MONDAY

Breakfast	1 C cooked grits
	1 C melon balls
Lunch	*Vegetable and tuna salad* (see recipe below)
	10 whole wheat crackers
	1 fresh orange
	calorie-free beverage
Dinner	1 oz whole wheat roll with 2 t reduced-fat margarine
	1 C cooked beets
	⅓ C white or brown rice with 1 t reduced-fat margarine
	3 oz roast chicken topped with mushrooms that have been simmered in giblet broth
	calorie-free beverage and salad

Vegetable and Tuna Salad

In a medium bowl blend 2 oz of tuna (canned in water) with ½ C cooked string beans, 1 small potato cooked and cut into large chunks, ¼ t parsley, ⅛ t powdered garlic, 1 chopped scallion (or 1 T coarsely chopped Bermuda onion) and 2 T reduced-fat salad dressing of your choice.

DAY 2 ■ TUESDAY

Breakfast 1¼ C corn flakes
8 oz 1% fat milk
4½ inches of sliced banana
coffee or tea

Lunch *Pita and cheese sandwich*
1 whole wheat pita bread (2 oz) filled with: 2 oz low-fat cheddar or mozzarella-style cheese in chunks, 4 cherry tomatoes (halved), ½ diced green pepper, and chunks of lettuce
2 T reduced-fat salad dressing of your choice
15 grapes
calorie-free beverage

Dinner 1 C cooked turnip greens seasoned with crushed red pepper and onions
¾ C mashed white potato and turnip blend, seasoned with 2 t reduced-fat margarine and 2 oz canned evaporated skimmed milk per serving
3 oz broiled pork chop
calorie-free beverage and salad
Baked apple (in place of 100-calorie dessert or snack)

Baked Apple

For each serving use 1 medium-large tart baking apple (such as Grannie Smith). Scoop out the core, leaving the apple whole. Place the apple(s) in a microwave-safe dish. If microwaving more than 1 apple, position them so that the center of the oven is vacant. Generously sprinkle cinnamon on top of the apple(s). Cover the apple(s) and bake in a microwave for approximately 4 minutes per apple or approximately 20 minutes in a regular oven.

DAY 3 ■ WEDNESDAY

Breakfast	1 bakery bran muffin
	⅔ C grapefruit sections
	6 oz 1% fat milk
	coffee or tea
Lunch	6 oz black bean soup
	Open-face salmon sandwich
	¼ C canned salmon, 1 slice of whole grain bread, topped with 3 t of reduced-fat mayonnaise, a sprinkle of dried basil, black pepper, and salt (optional)
	1 fresh pear
	calorie-free beverage
Dinner	1 C yellow squash, cooked
	¾ C cooked spinach noodles topped with 1 t reduced-fat margarine
	4 oz *oven-fried chicken*
	calorie-free beverage and salad

Oven-Fried Chicken

Prepare chicken pieces by dipping them first in slightly beaten egg white, then in seasoned bread crumbs (if you season your own, use fresh crumbs, a generous amount of dried parsley, oregano, Parmesan cheese, and salt to taste), then lightly spray the chicken with canola or other vegetable oil. Bake on a cookie sheet, without the pieces touching, at 350 degrees for 40 to 45 minutes or until golden brown.

DAY 4 ■ THURSDAY

Breakfast *Creamy and peachy oatmeal* with 4 oz canned evaporated skim milk
coffee or tea

Lunch *Turkey burger:*
2 oz ground turkey patty, 1 hamburger roll
carrot sticks
½ C string beans
calorie-free beverage

Dinner 1 C cauliflower sautéed with diced red and green bell pepper in 2 t regular margarine
⅔ C kernel corn
3 oz beef round, roasted in a covered pan with ½ inch of water and a sprinkle of dried dill weed
calorie-free beverage

Creamy and Peachy Oatmeal

In a medium saucepan, add 1 C of cold water, ½ C raw oatmeal (the one-minute cooking variety), 1 fresh peach or 2 dried peach halves, diced, and ¼ t of cinnamon. Bring it to a boil and cook one minute. Let it stand for several minutes. This is one serving.

DAY 5 ■ FRIDAY

Breakfast 1¼ C bran flakes
8 oz 1% fat milk
1¼ C fresh strawberries
coffee or tea

Lunch *Rainbow pasta salad* with 2 T of reduced-fat dressing (Take this to work in a spill-proof container.)
6 oz vegetable juice, served hot

	1 medium nectarine
	calorie-free beverage
Dinner	1 C kale, boiled
	1 baked sweet potato (approximately 5 inches long)
	5 oz turkey leg, roasted
	calorie-free beverage

Rainbow Pasta Salad

In a large bowl, combine 2 C of cooked corkscrew pasta or bow ties, ½ C coarsely chopped scallions, 1 C shredded red cabbage, ½ C celery that has been thinly sliced on the diagonal, ½ C coarsely grated carrots, ¾ C mandarin oranges (drained), and ¼ C slivered almonds or other chopped nuts (such as walnuts, pecans). One serving = ½ of dish.

DAY 6 ■ SATURDAY

Breakfast	1 English muffin with 2 t reduced-fat margarine
	¾ C orange sections
	1 egg prepared without fat
Lunch	1 slice of pizza from a 14-inch pie (⅛ of whole)
	cucumber spears
	calorie-free beverage
Dinner	*Chicken stew*
	calorie-free beverage and salad

Chicken Stew

In a large Dutch oven, brown ½ of a large onion and 1 clove of garlic (crushed) in 2 T of canola or other vegetable oil. Add 3 to 4 lbs chicken after removing skin and cutting meat into medium-sized pieces, 2 t parsley,

1 t rosemary, ½ t ground sage, ¼ t black pepper, and salt (optional) to taste. Add 1 C water and simmer for 20 minutes. Add a 10-oz box of frozen string beans, 4 raw carrots cut into chunks, and 4 large potatoes (peeled if desired) cut into chunks. Simmer for an additional 15 or 20 minutes or until all vegetables are firm but tender. One serving = ¼ of dish.

DAY 7 ■ SUNDAY

Breakfast
- 1 C cooked Cream of Wheat served with 2 t reduced-fat margarine
- 8 oz 1% fat milk
- 1 fresh nectarine
- coffee or tea

Dinner
- 1 C cooked collard greens
- 1 C *baked macaroni and cheese*
- 4 oz baked lean ham
- calorie-free beverage and salad

Supper
- 10 oz vegetable soup
- 2 slices whole wheat toast with 2 t reduced-fat margarine
- calorie-free beverage

Baked Macaroni and Cheese

In a large bowl, combine 1 slightly beaten egg, a 12 oz can of evaporated skimmed milk, 10 oz reduced-fat cheddar-style cheese, ¼ t black pepper, 1 t salt (optional), and 8 oz (raw weight) cooked elbow macaroni noodles. Pour into a lightly greased 2-quart baking dish and top with 2 oz grated cheese and paprika. Bake at 350 degrees for 25 minutes, or until lightly browned.

DAY 8 ■ MONDAY

Breakfast	1½ C puffed wheat 8 oz 1% fat milk 1 slice whole wheat toast served with 1½ t reduced-fat margarine 1 fresh pear, sliced coffee or tea
Lunch	*Tuna fish salad sandwich* 2 oz tuna (canned in water) and 1 T reduced-fat mayonnaise, 2 slices whole grain 40-calorie bread 10 French fries with 2 T catsup 1 C mixed fruit salad calorie-free beverage
Dinner	1 C steamed zucchini 1 C spaghetti with ½ C fat-free spaghetti sauce 2 oz lean ground beef or ground turkey (can be blended in the sauce or as meat balls) 2 T grated Parmesan cheese calorie-free beverage and salad

DAY 9 ■ TUESDAY

Breakfast	2 waffles (either frozen or homemade) ½ C applesauce, heated and served over the waffles coffee or tea
Lunch	*Bean salad* ½ tomato, ⅓ C mixed beans (kidney beans, chickpeas, etc.), 1 C assorted cooked vegetables, served with 2 T reduced-calorie dressing

	1 slice whole grain bread with 1 t reduced-fat margarine
	¼ medium cantaloupe
Dinner	1 C cooked spinach
	1 C cooked red potatoes
	Escovitch fish
	calorie-free beverage and salad

Escovitch Fish

Prepare about 1 lb of lean, fresh fish (such as cod, flounder, etc.) by sprinkling it with the juice of ½ large lemon or lime and black pepper. Set it aside. In a saucepan, blend 2 T canola or other vegetable oil, ⅓ C vinegar, 1 medium onion and 2 cloves of garlic (finely chopped by hand or in a food processor), 5 scallions, ⅛ t dried red pepper, 1 t salt (optional), ½ t dried all-spice, and ½ t crushed bay leaf. Bring these ingredients to a boil and keep hot. Bake the fish in a flat pan that is at least 2 inches deep at 350 degrees until the flesh is white. The length of time will depend on the thickness of the fish. When the fish is flaky, pour the liquid over the fish. This can be served hot or refrigerated and served cold. One serving = approximately ⅓ of dish.

DAY 10 ■ WEDNESDAY

Breakfast	1 C cooked grits served with 2 t reduced-fat margarine
	2 small fresh plums (or 3 canned plums)
	8 oz 1% fat milk
	coffee or tea
Lunch	1 bowl wonton soup (broth and one wonton)
	⅔ C white or brown rice

	1 C mixed steamed vegetables (such as broccoli, carrots, celery, etc.)
	½ C lean protein in chunks (such as shrimp, chicken, beef, etc.) mixed in with the vegetables
	⅓ C pineapple chunks
	calorie-free beverage
Dinner	*Curried peas and pasta*
	3 oz broiled chicken breast
	calorie-free beverage and salad

Curried Peas and Pasta

In a medium skillet, heat 2 t canola or other vegetable oil, add ½ t curry powder and salt (optional) to taste. Blend in 1 C of cooked sweet peas and 1 C cooked curly pasta or spaghetti and heat for approximately 3 minutes or until heated thoroughly. One serving = ½ of dish.

DAY 11 ■ THURSDAY

Breakfast	1¼ C shredded wheat
	3 stewed prunes
	8 oz 1% fat milk
	coffee or tea
Lunch	*Salad bar* (such as at a chain restaurant)
	¼ C tuna salad
	unlimited lettuce, green and red bell pepper, cucumber, radishes, cherry tomatoes, string beans
	⅓ C chickpeas (or other beans at the salad bar)
	2 T reduced-fat salad dressing
	2 bread sticks

	8 oz clear soup (such as consomme or low-fat beef onion)
	1 medium fresh orange
	calorie-free beverage
Dinner	1 C cooked mustard greens
	⅔ C white or brown rice
	3 oz *ground turkey meat loaf*
	calorie-free beverage and salad

Ground Turkey Meat Loaf

In a large bowl, blend 2 lbs ground turkey, ½ C seasoned bread crumbs, 1 slightly beaten egg (or ¼ C egg substitute), ½ C catsup, 3 T finely chopped onion, and salt and pepper to taste. Bake in a large (9-inch long) loaf pan at 350 degrees for 40 minutes. Let stand for 5 minutes before slicing.

DAY 12 ■ FRIDAY

Breakfast	1 English muffin
	2 t reduced-fat margarine
	½ large mango
	coffee or tea
Lunch	(Brown bag this sandwich and microwave at lunchtime.)
	Fish stick sandwich
	2½ oz fish sticks (select the low-fat varieties of frozen fish sticks in the supermarket)
	1 hamburger bun
	2 t mayonnaise or tartar sauce
	8 oz vegetable soup
	1 fresh peach
	calorie-free vegetables
Dinner	1½ C *shrimp gumbo*

served on ⅔ C white or brown rice
calorie-free beverage and salad

Shrimp Gumbo

In a large deep pot, sauté ½ C finely chopped onion in 2 T canola or other vegetable oil until translucent. Add 1 C water or chicken broth and 2 T dried thyme, and bring to boil. Add a 10-oz box of frozen lima beans and simmer for 6 minutes. Add a 10-oz box of frozen okra and simmer for 3 minutes. Add a 10-oz box of frozen corn and simmer for 3 minutes. Add 1-lb can of whole peeled tomatoes (slightly chopped) and 1 lb cleaned, deveined shrimp. Simmer for approximately 5 minutes or until shrimp turn red and mixture is hot throughout.

DAY 13 ■ SATURDAY

Breakfast 1 C cooked oatmeal sprinkled with cinnamon
1 kiwi, sliced
4 oz evaporated skimmed milk
coffee or tea

Lunch 2 C *vegetable medley*
2 x 2-in cube of corn bread (made with stone-ground cornmeal)
2 t reduced-fat margarine
1 fresh medium apple
calorie-free beverage

Dinner 1 C steamed broccoli
1 C cooked noodles
5 oz roasted pork
calorie-free beverage and salad

Vegetable Medley

In a large pot, sauté ½ C onion, 2 cloves garlic (minced), ¼ t black pepper, ¼ C diced green pepper, seasoning* and 2 stalks coarsely chopped celery. Add 1 C coarsely chopped mushrooms, 3 small quartered russet potatoes, 3 scraped and chunked carrots, ½ lb cleaned and halved string beans, and simmer for 20 minutes. Add 2 small cleaned zucchini that have been cut into ¾-in pieces and 1 can of whole skinless tomatoes that have been coarsely chopped. Let this mixture simmer for 10 minutes. Vegetables should be crisp but tender.

*For seasoning, vary ½ t of curry powder or chili powder, ⅛ t saffron, or commercial blends of "Soul Seasoning," "Italian Seasoning," or "Creole/Cajun Seasoning."

DAY 14 ■ SUNDAY

Breakfast	1¼ C whole wheat cereal
	8 oz 1% fat milk
	1 C diced honeydew melon
	coffee or tea
Dinner	1 C cabbage, cooked
	⅔ C *Hoppin' John*
	3 oz roast chicken
	½ C stuffing
	calorie-free beverage and salad
Supper	10 whole wheat crackers
	2 oz cold, cooked cod fish drizzled with 1 t olive oil
	sliced tomatoes
	1 medium peach
	calorie-free beverage

Hoppin' John

Soak 2 C of dried black-eyed peas according to package directions. Refrigerate while soaking. In a large pot or Dutch oven, sauté 2 T minced green pepper, 1 T dried thyme, 1 bay leaf, 1 large chopped onion, 1 chopped celery stalk, ¼ t black pepper, ½ t crushed red pepper, and salt to taste. For additional flavor you can add a smoked turkey wing. Add soaked beans and enough water to cover the beans in about 2 inches of water. Simmer for 2 hours, adding water to keep beans covered. Add 2 C uncooked brown rice to the pot; be sure there is no more than about 1 inch of water over the beans when you add the rice. (It is better to add a bit more water if the mixture is too dry.) Simmer for an additional 40 minutes and remove from heat. Keep pot tightly covered and let the steam complete the cooking and dry out the rice and bean mixture. If you do not use brown rice, use converted rice and cook for only 20 minutes before removing from heat. Keep the lid on until time to serve.

CHAPTER 9

Parting Thoughts

America is in the midst of what can only be described as a "fat revolution." Take medicine, for example. If you were overweight a generation or two ago, doctors pretty much shrugged their shoulders and assumed it was your own fault. Unfortunately, that view is still all too prevalent today. But what separates 1960 from the year 2000 is that scientists now have reason to believe that the tendency to become fat is inherited, even as they've also found compelling evidence that a sound eating plan and regular exercise can lead to better emotional and physical health and often some degree of permanent weight loss as well.

The future will continue to bring exciting revelations about body weight. Obesity researcher Dr. Jules Hirsch admits that such hopeful signs are a breath of fresh air. "For the last five to eight years, I was really in the doldrums," Hirsch told the *New York Times*, referring to the difficulty of helping severely obese patients lose weight and keep it off. "Prospects opened up by new techniques in biology have really raised my spirits."

For instance, in the years to come, geneticists will continue to contribute findings on what makes people fat. Scientists are cloning, or duplicating, the gene responsible for obesity in mice. From there, they hope to understand how the gene works and how the regulation of body weight in people differs from that in mice. The payoff may be a new appreciation for why and how people become fat. Once we understand how fat builds up, we may get a better handle on how to help people lose weight.

Clinical researchers may give us important clues to the types of weight-loss programs that work best for African-Americans. In the past, most participants in weight-loss trials have been white, even though the black population is substantially heavier. If there are differences in how blacks and whites lose weight, clinical trials with black folks will help us develop more effective weight-loss strategies for the community that needs it most.

Behavioral scientists may help us figure out how to best encourage black youngsters to stay healthy and prevent weight-related problems from developing. No black child wants to grow up sick, and none looks forward to an early death. But we don't always give our youngsters the information and hope that they need to stay healthy, sometimes because our own attitudes about health are tinged by fatalism. New research on health behavior and health attitudes may benefit African-Americans young and old alike.

Epidemiologists may help us develop weight standards that are more appropriate for African-Americans than are the standard life insurance tables. If we can understand the range of body weights that are the healthiest for black Americans, we can aim for more realistic weight goals based on African-Americans' own health experiences rather than standards based on white middle-class males.

Psychobiologists—scientists who specialize in the interaction between mental and biological processes—will contribute a new understanding about a phenomenon known as *seasonal affective disorder.* This mood alteration, marked by depression, anxiety, reduced sex drive, and increased appetite, stems from sunlight—or too little sunlight, to be precise. It affects most people, many of them women, for months at a time during the brief daylight of winter.

From pharmaceutical houses will come new medicines for weight loss. A generation ago, the most prominent weight-loss aid you could find was a stimulant that wasn't too effective and could do a number on your blood pressure. Nowadays, folks with stubborn weight problems can look forward to the development of a whole range of potential allies, including medicines that boost your metabolism, block fat from entering your system, or turn off your hunger switch.

The years ahead will undoubtedly continue to change how Americans feel about body weight, too. Discrimination against fat people will eventually go the way of racism and sexism, two social forces that are beginning (albeit haltingly) to become less socially acceptable. Black Americans who are overweight may be beneficiaries of the larger "fat liberation" movement, whose ultimate message of tolerance and equal opportunity meshes well with the respect that the African-American community has historically shown our heavier brothers and sisters. And that respect is important, because since slavery, African-Americans have known the value of believing in ourselves when no one else would. That same self-confidence carries us through today, no matter what our body size. You can hear it in the words of Sonskeshana Kornegay, secretary to Harlem's Congressman Charles Rangel, who was asked by an admiring *Ms.* magazine journalist how she manages to exude "the kind of personal magnetism that makes you want to follow her around and ask her to adopt you." Kornegay replied that her mother always made sure that she and her sister weren't ashamed of themselves, even though they were the biggest kids in the projects. "My mother would say, 'Hold your head up, straighten your shoulders, and be proud of who you are.' I carried that with me to adulthood."

At the same time, as more and more African-American youngsters, elders, and others in between understand the importance of fitness and good nutrition, and learn to take charge of our health, we will see more energetic efforts to prevent black people from getting fat and to encourage the heavier among us to slim down. It won't be that we consider our larger brothers and sisters any less deserving of respect. The concern will be for health. And the realization will be that while African-Americans currently bear the brunt of an amazing range of diseases and afflictions, it doesn't have to be that way. We don't have to die before our time.

So the trends affecting the African-American community may cut in two directions that may at first seem contradictory—on the one hand, self-acceptance for large people; on the other, concern for the health risks that obesity can symbolize. If there's a unifying principle here, it was coined by *Essence* magazine: "Large is lovely, unless you're unhappy, overeating, and unable to lose that weight." Or, we might add, unless your weight is hurting your health.

And if that's the case, know that there's hope. It's not easy to lose weight, at least not permanently. But what *is* within each of us is the ability to be healthier and to feel better about our bodies, and to inspire that same self-respect and self-love in our children and others. When we decide to make permanent, lifelong changes in our eating and exercising habits, we make that happen.

Much of the power lies within ourselves. All we need is a little guidance and encouragement to help us on our way. We hope this book gives you the boost to make that important first step to greater happiness and health.

Good luck and peace.

Glossary

"Apple" physique—a body shape marked by excess belly fat.

Autonomic nervous system—a part of the nervous system that controls metabolism, heartbeat, and other automatic functions.

Diastolic—blood pressure when the heart is at rest. It is the lower of the two blood pressure numbers.

Exchange list—a collection of foods with similar nutritional profiles.

Food diary—a personal record of the amount and type of food consumed, and location, mood, and hunger level during a meal or snack.

Gastric stomach bypass—surgery that attaches a section of the small intestine directly to the stomach to reduce the amount of nutrients absorbed by the body.

Hyperlipidemia—excess fats in the bloodstream.

Ideal weight—a range of body weights for a given height which are associated with the least amount of premature death.

Insulin—a hormone secreted by the pancreas and responsible for transporting glucose throughout the body.

Left ventricular hypertrophy—abnormal enlargement of the left ventricle, one of four heart chambers.

Liposuction—surgical suction of fat from the body.

Morbid obesity—twice a person's ideal weight, or 100 pounds over their ideal weight.

Nephron—a filtering tube, which produces urine, in the kidney.

Neurotransmitter—a chemical that allows nerves to communicate.

Obesity—clinically, 20 percent or more over a person's ideal weight.

Overweight—clinically, 10 to 20 percent over a person's ideal weight.

"Pear" physique—a body shape marked by excess fat on the thighs and buttocks.

Set point—a weight level to which the body returns after prolonged periods of too little or too much food intake.

Stomach stapling—surgical closure of much of the stomach to create a smaller chamber for food digestion.

Systolic—blood pressure when the heart is pumping. It is the higher of the two blood pressure numbers.

INDEX

About the Authors

MAVIS THOMPSON, M.D., is a retired family physician who for forty-five years has used nutrition and other holistic approaches in the prevention of illness. She is past president of the American Public Health Association's Black Caucus and a frequent speaker on topics ranging from teen nutrition to ethnic medical concerns.

KIRK A. JOHNSON is founding editor of the award-winning *Journal of Health Care for the Poor and Underserved,* published by Meharry Medical College in Nashville, Tennessee. He was senior researcher on the PBS civil-rights documentary "Eyes on the Prize," and has testified before Congress on health protection for minorities. His work appears in national publications such as *Heart & Soul, Essence, HealthQuest,* and *Columbia Journalism Review.*

LINDA VILLAROSA is an editor in the science department of the *New York Times* and former executive editor of *Essence* magazine. She is also the author of three books, including *Body & Soul: The Black Women's Guide to Physical Health and Emotional Well-Being.*

MAUDENE NELSON, M.S., R.D., a registered dietitian and certified diabetes educator, is a staff associate at the Institute of Human Nutrition, College of Physicians & Surgeons, Columbia University, and a nutritionist for the Arteriosclerosis Research Center at Columbia-Presbyterian Medical Center.